THE LUMBAR SPINE

MECHANICAL DIAGNOSIS AND THERAPY

R. A. McKenzie, O.B.E., F.C.S.P., F.N.Z.S.P. (HON), DIP. M.T.

SPINAL PUBLICATIONS
1981

SPINAL PUBLICATIONS LIMITED
P.O. BOX 93, WAIKANAE, WELLINGTON, NEW ZEALAND.

FIRST PRINTED 1981
REPRINTED 1981
REPRINTED 1982
REPRINTED 1983 (TWICE)
REPRINTED 1984
REPRINTED 1985
REPRINTED 1986
REPRINTED 1987
REPRINTED 1989
REPRINTED 1990
REPRINTED 1991
REPRINTED 1992

ISBN 0 473 00064 4

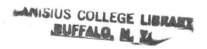
PRINTED BY WRIGHT & CARMAN LIMITED, UPPER HUTT, NEW ZEALAND

To my wife
Joy.

Acknowledgments

It is no coincidence that many of the statements in this book have a familiarity about them which traces back to the work of Dr James Cyriax. His influence has pervaded all mechanical spinal therapy, and his place as the father of orthopaedic medicine is unchallenged. I gratefully acknowledge the inspiration obtained from Cyriax which enabled me to develop some of his ideas, not necessarily in his fashion but, I am sure, in a manner of which he will approve.

My warmest thanks must go to Dr John Ebbetts who, early in my career, arranged for the international exposure of my treatment method for acute lumbar scoliosis.

I am most grateful to the doctors of Wellington, New Zealand, who have supported me over the past twenty-eight years. Without their confidence and encouragement the development of these concepts and treatment methods would not have been possible.

I thank Dr Arthur White of San Francisco for contributing the Foreword to this book and for giving me the opportunity to demonstrate to him, the effectiveness of the methods described within.

To Dr Edward Miller, Professor of Orthopaedics at University of Cincinatti Medical Center, to the physical therapists, physicians and orthopaedic surgeons of the Kaiser Permanente Medical Centres of California, I am greatly indebted for support and backing that has led to wide acceptance of my ideas throughout the United States.

My former assistant Glen Pendergrast must be held responsible for me putting pen to paper, as he casually enquired who would know my work properly if I were run over by a bus. I appreciate his stimulation and support.

Finally, I sincerely thank my present assistant Paula Van Wijmen for the compilation of the information presented in this book. She is one of the very few people who, besides myself, fully understand these concepts. Without her knowledge, loyalty and perserverance this book would still be a notebook.

R. McKENZIE

Foreword

I am very pleased to present a foreword and commentary to this book by Mr McKenzie. It is a refreshing publication which I favour for several reasons.

First, the underlying thesis for this book is that the great majority of disabilities of the lumbar spine are mechanical, and thus can be treated in a mechanical manner. More important than that, once the principles are understood most of the mechanical treatments can be accomplished by the patient himself. In fact, the very goal of treatment as proposed by Mr McKenzie is to place the patient on a self care programme so that he will not require the care of therapists or medical clinicians. The mechanical abnormalities and postural variations are incurable, but at least if appropriate principles are understood, the majority of disability related to these can be avoided.

The second reason I favour this publication is its unpretentious flavour. The author recognises that physicians and surgeons seldom are interested or adept at the mechanical approach to physical disability. This is an area where therapists truly are adept, and by experience and training remain interested in the subject. On the other hand, there is very little scientific basis for our current understanding of the principles of care of the spine. Thus, to place a treatment programme on a level of scientific security which should be the ideal of medical treatment, is inappropriate. The author takes the position that the principles advocated in this text work on the majority of people, and the rationale for their success can only be presumed on a logical progression of our current level of knowledge. The programme is safe, inexpensive and indeed, may be scientifically accurate. Certainly the concepts proposed are as reliable and secure as any other conceptual framework used today in our understanding of chronic back disability.

I suppose the reason I really enjoyed the book most is that the author has taken a new tack in the analysis and treatment of the problem. He has shown an appropriate disrespect for "accepted principles". Only by the constant questioning of previously accepted truths will progress be made toward more complete understanding. Certainly many of the accepted principles of the past, such as the avoidance of lumbar extension, have not diminished the problem of chronic back disability which currently fills the offices of clinicians around the world. Lets try this new approach which has as rational a base as any of our treatments for clinical syndromes. It certainly is more rational than the use of various modalities such as ultrasound and various pharmacologic agents which try to solve the problem of local mechanical problems by systemic alterations in nervous system response. Anything that costs less, is not health threatening, and fixes most of the problems deserves a respected place in the medical treatment programmes. I am pleased that Mr McKenzie has chosen to stay within the mainstream of medicine and allied health professionals rather than to escape the scrutiny of cautious peers which has allowed many a flimsy fad to come and go. I expect the programme outlined by Mr McKenzie to grow in significance and acceptance as more people try it and benefit from it.

Vert Mooney, M.D.

Robin McKenzie has had a great influence on my treatment of low back pain. It was quite by accident that he and I lectured at the same low back pain seminar several years ago. Even though we had differing philosophies in regard to the etiology and treatment of low back pain, there was so much in common between us that I began a thorough scientific study of his techniques. I have found that twenty percent of my patient population are much more responsive to his methods than to any of the methods I have used in the past. My patient population is more of a chronic multi-operated back population and has generally speaking, resisted all previous therapies. In populations where the patients are seen early in their disease with acute injuries, I feel that fifty to eighty percent would be rapidly relieved by the techniques described in this book.

It is all too easy for those of us in the clinical profession to shun new techniques which do not fit our model of how medicine should be practised. I was fortunate enough to be introduced to Robin McKenzie during a period of professional growth in which I felt a need for a better understanding of the diagnosis and treatment of low back pain. The understanding of the McKenzie techniques has allowed me to improve the diagnosis and treatment of low back pain in my orthopaedic practice.

Information contained in the pages of this book works. I cannot substantiate, nor do I believe anyone can substantiate the exact reasons why it works. Robin McKenzie has some very appealing explanations for why his methods work. I only know for certain that they do work in a very busy orthopaedic and physical therapy spine centre in San Francisco.

I believe that this volume is one of the more important contributions to the literature on the treatment of low back pain and we will continue attempting to scientifically prove how well the McKenzie method works and the reason for its working. In addition to all of the above considerations, this book is enjoyable, as is the author.

Arthur H. White, M.D.
San Francisco.

Contents

Introduction

The treatment of low back pain remains as controversial today as it was fifty years ago. Over the years the medical profession used a wide range of treatments, such as heat or cold, rest or exercise, flexion or extension, mobilisation or immobilisation, manipulation or traction. Nearly always drugs were prescribed, even when the disturbance proved purely mechanical in origin. Amazingly, most of the patients recovered, very often in spite of treatment rather than because of it.

It is not surprising that the first half of this century found osteopaths and chiropractors in the forefront of those dispensing the most satisfactory treatments, at least as far as patients were concerned. Mechanical disturbances of the articular system are best treated by mechanical means. It is for this reason that unorthodox operators were more successful than the medical profession, because only few medical practitioners were capable of applying mechanical treatment.

We have to thank osteopathy and chiropractic for providing the stimulus required to move medicine in the right direction. Beginning with James Mennell and James Cyriax that momentum is gathering strength and, at present, understanding of the mechanics of low back pain is emanating from clinics and laboratories throughout the world.

There has been a trend in manipulative therapy to meekly follow in the footsteps of osteopaths and chiropractors. This is unlikely to produce significant and rapid improvement in spinal therapy. Many of the procedures and techniques presented by the early manipulators for treatment of mechanical spinal pain are valid, but only when applied to patients with certain well defined signs and symptoms. Manipulative procedures, already suspect in many cases, have a definite but limited application, and it is now clear which patients benefit from manipulation and which do not. Furthermore, it is likely that as our understanding improves, patients will require less rather than more manipulative procedures.

There has been a tendency among exponents of mobilisation and manipulation to overclaim and exaggerate the benefits to be derived from its administration. This trend must cease if we wish scientific development of mechanical therapy to proceed.

Most treatments appear to be directed at pain relief for the present episode. Episodic relief by therapy of any kind makes the patient dependent on that therapy and thereafter he will seek a quick answer for what is essentially a life-long problem. Whenever his back pain recurs he must attend a physician, manipulative therapist, chiropractor or osteopath. I believe that treatment dependency is undesirable and should be avoided where possible. Therefore, in addition to whatever treatment is necessary for present symptoms *the patient should be taught to become self-reliant and independent of therapists in the management of future low back pain.*

It is often thought that all patients presenting for treatment must have a pathological condition. I suggest to those peering down a microscope to find a pathological cause for mechanical joint pain, and to those seeking to provide a wonder drug for low back pain that, in its simplest form, low back pain starts for the same reason as pain arises in the forefinger when it is bent backwards far enough to stimulate the free nerve endings of periarticular structures. *No pathology needs to exist, and no chemical treatment will cure this form of mechanical pain.*

In this book I hope to explain clearly that there is a time when the low back should be extended and a time when it should be flexed; that there are circumstances when both procedures should be applied; and, perhaps most important of all, that it is now possible to identify in advance those patients who will respond to manipulation.

I have developed a simple classification: mechanical pain may develop from postural stresses; it may be the result of joint derangement or it may be caused by dysfunction. In patients with pure postural pain no pathology is present, and all that is required in their treatment is adequate explanation of the cause of pain and instruction in self-treatment by postural correction. In the majority of patients with joint derangement and dysfunction the pathological condition can be successfully influenced by mechanical therapy using the patient's own movements. A method of self-treatment and self-manipulation of the articular system is now available to patients who have enough understanding to learn and carry out the required procedures. In this book I intend to explain why self-treatment procedures are preferable to procedures that must be applied by a therapist.

Successful application of the self-treatment concept depends on the correct selection of patients. Throughout this book the assumption has been made that patients are referred for therapy by their doctor. Indeed, we require our medical practitioners to provide us with the appropriate patients — that is, patients who do not suffer from serious pathology (mechanical or other) and who have had all but mechanical causes of low back pain excluded. I hope that this book will enable the clinician to select from the people with low back pain those who may respond to mechanical treatment, and to place them in the three relatively simple categories. Once the appropriate syndrome is exposed the application of simple and inexpensive procedures, usually through the patient's own efforts, may effect cure. I believe that we can now identify those patients who may become self-reliant (seventy percent) and those who will always require some assistance from a therapist (thirty percent).

It is not necessary, indeed it is impossible, for the majority of doctors to keep abreast with modern developments in mechanical therapy. Consequently, not many doctors have the knowledge to prescribe specific treatments for patients with low back pain. As it is the responsibility of the therapist to maintain his knowledge and techniques in the field of mechanical therapy at the highest possible level, he is best able to define which type of treatment is most suitable for a particular mechanical problem. Thus, the choice of treatment lies with the therapist.

With this book I present a new concept of diagnosis for the whole musculo-skeletal system. The procedures I developed for the lumbar spine to arrive at appropriate conclusions regarding diagnosis and treatment, may also be applied successfully to the thoracic and cervical spine, and indeed to all peripheral joints and their surrounding soft tissues. Irrespective of the presenting pathology, the principles of diagnosis and treatment remain the same.

Having developed a method for treating low back pain that appears to work very well, it is incumbent on me to offer an explanation suggesting why these procedures are effective. I have hypothesised using mans present knowledge of the structure function and behaviour of the lumbar intervertebral discs. No proof absolute exists to substantiate this hypothesis but I believe it to be somewhere near the truth. Only time and much research will reveal the true nature of the mechanism responsible for the production of recurrent low back pain, but the influence of these procedures on that mechanism will be just as effective in fifty years time as they are today.

I have chosen to ignore many well accepted and established procedures, for after twenty seven years of clinical experience I must conclude that at best some of these are ineffective and at worst, injurious. We must constantly search for better methods to relieve pain and restore function and we will not progress if we repeat the procedures that have become established. Only by departing from the old pathway will we discover the new. It is my belief that we have merely scratched the surface and are in the embryonic stages of developing therapy for the musculo-skeletal system.

CHAPTER 1

Definition and Selection

Epidemiology

The frequency of back pain is such that in the United States alone there are seven million people off work because of it at any one time.[1] It is impossible to tell how many of these people suffer from low back pain but as it causes more lost time in industry than any other problem, the number must be impressive.

Figures obtained from the United Kingdom show that 1.1 million people aged fifteen and over consult their general practitioner in any one year for low back pain, and 13.2 million working days are lost because of low back pain.[2] Elsewhere is reported that back pain accounts for sixty-three percent of sickness absence in manual workers currently employed and probably causes the loss of more than fifteen million man-days per annum.[3]

Low back pain is the commonest cause of occupational disability in industrial societies and, with headache, is the most frequent variety of pain with which general practitioners have to contend.[4] From an extensive study[5] it appears that significant low back pain begins at the age of about thirty-five. The same study reveals that of the total number of people examined thirty-five percent would get sciatica, and ninety percent would become recurrent.

Low back pain is not necessarily a consequence of degenerative processes for many patients with recurring low back pain have no evidence of degenerative changes, and many people who do have degenerative radiological changes have no back pain. It is clearly stated[6] that there is no obvious relationship between degenerative changes and low back pain. Furthermore, x-rays of well known weight lifters show no relationship between radiological changes and the ability to perform heavy work.[5]

The occupational incidence of low back pain is described by Nachemson:[7]

"Low back pain occurs with about the same frequency in people with sedentary occupations as in those doing heavy labour, although the latter have a higher incidence of absence from work because they are unable to work with their complaint".

It follows that a common denominator must exist in the production of low back pain. If physical exertion is not a predominant factor, there must be some inherent faults in our lifestyle to cause such a widespread problem. The great majority of patients with low back pain state that they have increased pain while sitting or on arising from sitting. It is my belief that almost all low back pain is

1

aggravated and perpetuated, if not caused, by poor sitting postures in both sedentary and manual workers.

The enormous cost incurred by a society bearing the responsibility for care, treatment and rehabilitation of people with low back pain is overshadowed by the problems of human disability and suffering, experienced not only by those directly affected but also by their immediate families.

Self-limitation

All practitioners within and without the orthodox medical field are assured of excellent results in the treatment of many disorders, including low back pain, because of the self-limiting nature of many human ills. Statistics have shown that fourty-four percent of patients with low back pain are better in one week, eighty-six percent within one month, and ninety-two percent within two months.[8] So, the manipulator who continues to adjust the spine for about eight weeks is assured of a ninety-two percent success rate. An equally good result can be obtained by applying a heat lamp for a similar period of time, or by doing precisely nothing.

If the problems surrounding low back pain were as simple as that, there would be little need for clinicians and therapists to devote so much time to its treatment. However, the difficulties do not lie in treating a particular episode of low back pain but more in the prevention of future episodes. From my own figures it appears that about sixty-two percent of patients attending for treatment have had episodic pain on at least three occasions in the past five years.

Although self-limiting, low back pain will often recur and the recurrences tend to become progressively more severe with each successive attack. If we are to succeed in reducing the incidence of recurrent low back pain, we must aim our treatments at patient education and teaching of prophylactic methods. It is my practise to teach patients to stop their own pain, and this can only be done when that pain is present. Therefore, treatment must be implemented during an attack of low back pain rather than after it has subsided. A patient who has no pain at present cannot be taught effectively to stop pain when it next appears. For this reason a good case exists for treatment early in an episode of low back pain, despite the automatic recovery that can generally be expected.

Definition and selection

Most likely to respond to my treatment methods are patients suffering from low back pain, which is defined by Nachemson[7] as follows:

"Acute, sub-acute or chronic low back pain, which is characterised by either a slowly or a suddenly occurring rather sharp pain with or without radiation over the buttocks or slightly down the leg, and concomitant restriction of motion. When subsiding to the chronic type, the pain will be a little less severe and continue for more than two months."

Often these patients describe recurrent symptoms, and a recurrent episodic history is a common feature of the low back pain syndrome.

In addition to patients with low back pain as described above it is important to include the patients who have *intermittent sciatica without neurological deficit,* for many of these can successfully be treated as well. However, the intermittency must be a truly intermittent phenomenon — that is, there must be times in the day when the patient feels neither sciatic pain nor paraesthesiae.

I exclude the patients in whom no position or movement can be found to reduce or centralise pain patterns. Patients who have truly *constant severe sciatica with neurological deficit* are, in my opinion, unsuited to any mechanical procedure other than perhaps traction applied while on bed rest. This is not to suggest they will remain unsuitable. Reassessment at the end of a week or two is probably appropriate.

It may well be that a patient without sciatica has such intense pain in the back that he cannot be treated immediately. After one to two days of bedrest in the correct position he must be reassessed and may be found suitable for treatment.

I rely on my referring medical practitioners to exclude all patients with serious and unsuitable pathologies, but occasionally a patient with low back pain of non-mechanical origin will slip through the sieve. We must be aware that this may happen and, provided we use mechanical diagnostic procedures and carefully assess the patients response to treatment we will always detect mistakes of this nature.

CHAPTER 2

Predisposing and Precipitating Factors

PREDISPOSING FACTORS

Sitting posture

There are three predisposing factors in the etiology of low back pain that overshadow most others. The first and most important factor is the sitting posture. A good sitting posture maintains the spinal curves normally present in the erect standing position. Postures which reduce or accentuate the normal curves enough to place the ligamentous structures under full stretch will eventually be productive of pain. Such postures are referred to as poor sitting postures.

A poor sitting posture may *produce* back pain in itself without any additional other strains of living.[9, 10] We have all seen patients who entered an airliner, a car, or even a common lounge chair in a perfectly healthy and painfree state only to emerge hours later crippled with pain and unable to walk upright.

Alternatively, a poor sitting posture will frequently *enhance and always perpetuate* the problems in patients suffering from low back pain. By far the great majority of patients complain of an increase in pain *while sitting or on rising from sitting*. On examination of thousands of patients, many of them in Europe and North America, the same picture emerges: those people who are developing low back pain problems nearly always have a poor sitting posture.

As Wyke[4] has said, once a person has been sitting in a chair for more than a few minutes the lumbar spine assumes the fully flexed position. In this position the musculature is relaxed and the weight bearing strains are absorbed by the ligamentous structures. Try the following experiment yourself: sit relaxed in any chair and think of nothing in particular; after ten minutes deliberately try to produce more flexion in the low back; very little will happen. Without you realising it your spine has fallen into full flexion. *Relaxed sitting for any length of time places the lumbar spine in a fully stretched position.* This will become painful, if maintained for a prolonged period.

By sitting in this manner we are repeatedly doing to our low back something we would not permit to happen in any extremity joint. We do not hold our wrist, ankle, knee or shoulder in a fully stretched position until or after it has become painful. Instead, when the stress exceeds a certain limit the position of

4

the limb is automatically changed from the fully stretched position. A similar but less effective mechanism applies to the low back in sitting: when pain arises while sitting we merely change from one position of full stretch to another.

In general, relaxed sitting tends to become a poor sitting posture. It is difficult to avoid stress on the lumbar spine in relaxed sitting unless special instructions are followed. There is little hope of curing low back pain as long as our patients are permitted to sit incorrectly.

Andersson et al.[11] have demonstrated how in sitting the intradiscal pressure increases as the spine moves into kyphosis, and decreases as it moves into lordosis. Clinically, patients often describe that during sitting their pain increases with movement towards kyphosis and decreases with movement towards lordosis. In these instances there is a correlation between intradiscal pressure and pain patterns which may well incriminate the intervertebral disc as being responsible for, or at least contributing to, the production of low back pain.

Environmental factors may contribute greatly to the etiology of low back pain due to sitting. Working platforms which are not adjusted to individual requirements, and poorly designed seating for domestic, commercial and transportation purposes will promote poor sitting postures. Expensive anthropometric and ergonomic studies, aimed at improving office furniture, have failed to produce the desired result in respect of adequate support and comfort for the low back. A re-design of furniture may be necessary, based on the concepts of efficient working positions in sitting. Unless pressure can be brought to bear on manufacturers of seating furniture, poorly designed chairs will continue to add to the misery of patients with low back pain. In the meantime we should educate our young and re-educate the rest of the community regarding the correct sitting posture, for even the best designed chairs will be used incorrectly unless the user understands what is the correct position.

Postural factors other than sitting may predispose to low back pain. Some sleeping positions and work-related postures may be potentially damaging and will under certain circumstances cause or perpetuate low back pain. Such factors are not discussed here. However, they should be kept in mind and dealt with individually as they present themselves.

Loss of extension range

The second factor predisposing to the production of low back pain and its recurrence is the loss of lumbar extension. Studies in 1972[12] and 1979[10] indicated that respectively seventy-five and eighty-six percent of patients with low back pain had a loss of extension. A reduced range of extension influences the posture in sitting, standing and walking.

As a result of poor postural habits especially in affluent societies man gradually loses the ability to perform certain movements. From postural causes alone the lumbar spine undergoes adaptive changes and from my own observations it appears that few adults reach thirty years of age and maintain normal extension movements. The loss is reversible (with effort) up to fifty or sixty years of age in many patients.

If low back pain has been evident in the patients previous history, there is nearly always some modest restriction of lumbar extension which will improve if the appropriate exercising is commenced. I believe in these patients the loss of extension is caused by bad posture or lack of adequate movement at the time that repair mechanisms were operative. As healing occurs, adaptive shortening of scar tissue prevents movement and unless the patient is adequately advised, the scarring will form with the spine held in the slightly flexed relaxed position, for few patients rest with the spine extended. Again it is the movement towards extension that remains limited.

A reduced range of extension acquired in either manner described, rarely recovers spontaneously to the full. Unless the patient takes specific measures to regain it, extension remains reduced and the ability to sit with a lordosis is impaired or lost.[10] It is not generally recognised that it is impossible to sit and maintain a lordosis without an adequate extension range. Patients who, for some reason or other, have to sit with a flattened lumbar spine, are condemned to sit with a raised intradiscal pressure as well as a taut posterior annular wall.

Reduced extension is not only an impediment to the adoption of good sitting postures, it is also a major obstruction to obtaining the fully upright posture in standing. A reduced extension range will produce full stretch positions prematurely during prolonged and relaxed standing, and once sufficient stress is present, pain will arise.

As the loss of extension increases, the patient will be forced to walk slightly stooped. The maintenance of the slightly flexed posture creates a constant stress on the nucleus and posterior annular wall. Under normal circumstances this stress is relieved by moving into extension. However, as extension is no longer possible lasting relief cannot be obtained. Eventually adaptive changes will extend to all periarticular structures including the apophyseal joints.

Frequency of flexion

The third predisposing factor to low back pain is the frequency of flexion. When one examines the lifestyle of western cultures in the twentieth century, it is not hard to understand why man is losing his ability to freely extend the spine. He wakes in the morning, stoops over a wash basin and sits to have breakfast; all so far in flexion. He then travels to work by bus, train or car; he works bent forwards either in sitting or in standing; almost the whole day is spent in flexion. He sits travelling home, and again for his meal; then he may work in the garden or watch television for the evening, remaining flexed for most of the time. He sleeps in a flexed position nearly the whole night, awaking the next morning to repeat the cycle. It can safely be claimed that the spine is constantly being flexed to the maximum, but is rarely extended to the maximum.

When evaluating these predisposing factors it appears beneficial to recommend that patients with low back pain should extend the lumbar spine from time to time and under certain circumstances yet to be defined. This will theoretically reduce the stress on the posterior annular wall and simultaneously cause the fluid nucleus to move anteriorly — that is, away from the site of most protrusions and extrusions.[13, 14] Moreover, patients should sit with the lumbar spine supported in some extension as in this position the intradiscal pressure is reduced.[11, 15] The sensible use of extension to overcome the disadvantages of prolonged flexion seems to be a simple and logical step towards reducing some of the predisposing factors involved in low back pain and its recurrence. Here we have the *beginning of a prophylactic concept.*

Insufficient understanding of the mechanics involved in the production of low back pain has led some people to condemn extension of the spine and those who advocate it. If a Higher Authority had decided that extension is undesirable or harmful, the facet joints in the spine would have been placed accordingly! In the absence of such an indication it appears impertinent for man to place such restrictions on the use of the human frame, which after all has evolved over millions of years to become the wonderful, dynamic, mechanically bewildering and self-repairing marvel that it is. It managed to do this, I must add, without the benefits of medical specialisation.

PRECIPITATING FACTORS

The predisposing factors for low back pain and its recurrence are mostly related to positions and the short and long term consequences of maintaining them. Movement and activity may precipitate low back pain and therefore contribute to its incidence and recurrence.

Movements

It is often the unexpected and unguarded movement that causes a sudden episode of low back pain. This may occur during work related activities, be it domestic or occupational, and in sports and recreational activities — for example, squash, tennis, golf, football and gymnastics. Whatever the situation, when any of the predisposing factors are present very little is required to precipitate a sudden onset of low back pain, and the exciting strain may be an event as trivial as stooping momentarily.[12] When attempting to reduce the frequency of low back pain episodes, it is necessary to examine and advise each patient individually regarding the precipitating circumstances involved in his particular case.

Lifting

Lifting produces a strain which is often a precipitating factor, especially when heavy, prolonged and repeated lifting are involved. The risks of incurring low back pain are greater when the weight of the load to be lifted increases, and when lifting is performed by untrained and unfit people.[9]

Nachemson[16] describes the effects on the intradiscal pressure when certain positions are adopted while weights are held in the hands. Lifting from the forward bent position is one of the most stressful activities: when a certain weight is lifted with the back bent and the knees straight, the intradiscal pressure rises up to five times compared with that present when standing erect; however, when the same weight is lifted with the back straight and the knees bent there is a marked reduction in intradiscal pressure.

The coach of the Canadian Olympic weight lifting team explained to me that his team members were instructed to lift with a hollow in the low back. This he said prevented low back problems among the weight lifting fraternity.

Correct lifting techniques do have an effect on pain brought about by lifting. The more the lordosis is maintained while lifting, the less discomfort will be experienced. When appropriate, correct lifting should be taught as a prophylactic measure.

CHAPTER 3

The Cause of Pain

THE NOCICEPTIVE RECEPTOR SYSTEM

Most tissues in the body possess a system of nerve endings which, being particularly sensitive to tissue dysfunction, may be referred to as nociceptive receptors.[4] The free nerve endings of the nociceptive system provide the means by which we are made aware of pain.

Wyke[4] describes the distribution of the nociceptive receptor system in the lumbar area: it is found in the skin and subcutaneous tissue; throughout the fibrous capsule of all the synovial apophyseal joints and sacro-iliac joints; in the longitudinal ligaments, the flaval and interspinous ligaments and sacro-iliac ligaments; in the periosteum covering the vertebral bodies and arches, and in the fascia, aponeuroses and tendons attached thereto; and also in the spinal dura mater, including the dural sleeves surrounding the nerve roots.

The nociceptive innervation of the spinal ligaments varies from one ligament to another. The system is found to be most dense in the posterior longitudinal ligament, less in the anterior longitudinal ligament and sacro-iliac ligaments, and least in the flaval and interspinous ligaments.[4] This would suggest, that the posterior longitudinal ligament is more sensitive than the anterior ligament, and that the flaval and interspinous ligaments are least sensitive of all. Irrespective of this suggestion it is significant that the ligament which is most richly endowed with free nerve endings, is situated immediately adjacent to the only vital structures in the area — that is, the nerve roots and the spinal cord.

Although there is disagreement on the topic, Wyke states that the intervetebral disc contains no free nerve endings either in the nucleus or in the annulus. However, there are some nerve endings in the fibro-adipose tissue, that binds the posterior longitudinal ligament to the posterior portion of the annulus. Wyke[4] states:

"The only place where a nociceptive receptor system is directly related to the intervertebral discs is at the point where the discs (through the annulus fibrosus) are attached to the posterior longitudinal ligament; and the receptor system is not, in fact, in the disc itself, but in the surrounding connective tissue that links the disc to the posterior longitudinal ligament."

The wide distribution of the nociceptive receptor system in the lumbar area would make it difficult to devise testing procedures which selectively stress individual components of the spinal segments.

Mechanism of pain production

Again I must quote Wyke[4] who states that there are only two possible causes of pain. The following concept is most fundamental and essential in the understanding of the mechanism of pain production:

> "In normal circumstances this receptor system (that is, the nociceptive receptor system — Author's addition) is relatively (although not entirely) inactive; but its afferent activity is markedly enhanced when its constituent unmyelinated fibres are depolarised by the application of mechanical forces to the containing tissues that sufficiently *stress, deform or damage* (Author's italics) it (as with pressure, distraction, distension, abrasion, contusion or laceration) or by their exposure to the presence in the surrounding tissue fluid of sufficient concentration of irritating chemical substances that are released from traumatised, inflamed, necrosing or metabolically abnormal (and especially ischaemic) tissues."

Chemical cause of pain

Pain is produced by chemical irritation as soon as the concentration of chemical substances is sufficient to irritate free nerve endings in the involved soft tissues. This is of lesser interest to us as it encompasses either inflammatory or infective processes, such as active rheumatoid arthritis, ankylosing spondylitis, tuberculous and other bacterial infections. However, it also occurs in the first ten to twenty days following trauma. This will be discussed later.

Mechanical cause of pain

Pain is produced by the application of mechanical forces as soon as the mechanical deformation of structures containing the nociceptive receptor system is sufficient to irritate free nerve endings. It is not necessary to actually *damage* tissues containing the free nerve endings in order to provoke pain. Pain will also be produced by the application of forces sufficient to *stress or deform* the ligamentous and capsular structures. Pain will disappear when the application of that force is terminated, and this often occurs by a mere change of position. A good example is the pain, incurred during prolonged sitting which disappears on standing up.

Another simple example of mechanical articular pain is readily at hand. Bend your left forefinger backwards, using your right forefinger to apply overpressure. Keep applying this pressure until the nociceptive receptor system indicates its enhanced active state by the arrival of pain. This is simple mechanical deformation of pain sensitive structures. If you bend the finger backwards further, the intensity of the pain will increase; and if you maintain the painful position longer, the pain will become more diffuse, widespread and difficult to define. Thus, pain alters with increasing and prolonged mechanical deformation. If you now slowly return the finger to its normal resting position, the pain will disappear. This example has one significant implication: the finger is obviously being moved in the wrong direction as the pain increases, and in the correct direction as the pain decreases.

When the finger is used as an example the mechanism of pain production is easy to understand. But the same idea applied to the spine is more difficult to accept. In the spine the same mechanism is involved, but there are more structures which may give rise to pain and the mechanics are more complicated.

Let us return to the forefinger once more. Bend the finger backwards until you feel pain and then release it suddenly. The pain ceases at once. What was the pathology in the finger at the moment the pain appeared? What is the pathology now that the stress is released? Of course, the answer is that *no pathology need exist* at all under these circumstances. The sensation of pain does not depend on the existence of pathology. The example cited above is one of the most common causes of articular pain in man. The intermittent pain was produced by mechanical forces sufficient to stress or deform the nociceptive receptor system; the activity of the system was merely enhanced by the application of the stress, and as soon as the stress was withdrawn the activity returned to its normal rest level. Intermittent low back pain is frequently caused in this manner. No chemical treatment will rectify or prevent pain arising from mechanical deformation. When intermittent mechanical pain is the main presenting symptom, drugs should never be the treatment of choice, except in the presence of *extreme* pain.

Trauma as a cause of pain

Pain due to trauma is produced by a combination of mechanical deformation and chemical irritation. Initially, mechanical deformation causes damage to soft tissues, and pain of mechanical origin will be felt. In most instances this is a sharp pain. When in the lumbar spine mechanical deformation is severe enough to traumatise soft tissues, it is usually the result of an external force — for example, a fall from a ladder, a motor vehicle accident, a sudden unexpected step from the pavement, or a kick in the back during football.

Shortly after injury, chemical substances accumulate in the damaged tissues. As soon as the concentration of these chemical irritants is sufficient to enhance the activity of the nociceptive receptor system in the surrounding tissues, pain will be felt. In most instances pain of chemical origin will be experienced as a persistent discomfort or dull aching *as long as the chemicals are present in sufficient quantities*. In addition, the chemical irritants excite the nociceptive receptor system in such a way that the application of relatively minor stresses causes pain which under normal circumstances would not occur. Thus, at this stage there is a *constant pain, possibly a mild aching only, which may be enhanced but will never reduce or cease due to positioning or movement*.

The reaction of the body to trauma is to institute processes of repair, and the application of mechanical treatment should not be so vigorous as to delay healing. I believe that strenuous mechanical therapy in the presence of constant chemical pain merely delays recovery, and if the condition appears to improve while such treatment is given, improvement must take place in spite of it.

Over a period of five to twenty days healing occurs slowly and develops with the passage of time. Relative immobilisation of the damaged structures allows scarring to take place, and as scarring increases the concentration of chemical irritants decreases. In the later stages of healing when movements are performed more willingly, dysfunction caused by contraction and adaptive shortening of scar tissue will be exposed. Thus, after two to three weeks the *constant pain due to chemical irritation will have disappeared and is replaced by intermittent pain felt when adaptively shortened tissues are stretched.*

Causes of mechanical deformation

Mechanical deformation is caused by mechanical stress which, when applied to soft tissues, will lead to pain under certain circumstances. The following situations are possible:

— *Normal stress applied to normal tissue* will not *immediately* produce pain.
— *Abnormal stress applied to normal tissue* may produce pain without causing damage. This occurs in pure postural pain. Postural stresses, although normal when applied for short periods, become abnormal when sustained for long periods. Abnormal stress applied to normal tissue and resulting in damage will produce pain. This occurs in trauma.
— *Normal stress applied to abnormal tissue* will produce pain. The normal stress of the end range of movement, although painless in normal tissues, becomes painful in the presence of tissue abnormalities, especially in adaptive shortening.
— *Abnormal stress applied to abnormal tissue* will produce pain — for example, prolonged bending or sitting applied to adaptively shortened scar tissue may readily distort the tissue and be productive of pain. Reversal of the stressful position will result in reduction of pain. A similar stress applied to normal tissue is much less likely to cause pain.

Mechanical stresses sufficient to cause pain are usually created either by postural distortion or by abnormal forces applied to the stationary or moving body.

Postural stresses:

These are, according to Wyke,[4] by far the most often encountered and their importance is generally underestimated:

"Thus, although the fact has been demonstrated repeatedly over the past twenty-five years, it is still not sufficiently appreciated by the generality of doctors that much of the static postural support for the lower spine in the erect, sitting and fully flexed positions of the body is provided by the passive elastic tension of the ligaments and aponeuroses attached thereto, rather than by neurologically-engendered motor unit activity in the paravertebral musculature. As these connective tissues are richly innervated by nociceptive nerve endings, it will be clear that backache is readily produced from these tissues when they are subjected to abnormal mechanical stresses (as by prolonged standing, especially while wearing high heeled shoes; by persistantly distorted postures in occupational circumstances, or as a result of structural abnormalities of the vertebral column; or by attempts to lift or support heavy weights), or when their elasticity is decreased (as it inevitably is with advancing age, or as a result of hormonal changes)".

When a relaxed position is assumed for more than a few minutes, the muscular control required to hold the individual in that particular position diminishes, the body sags and the support is derived from the ligaments. Essentially the muscles relax slowly in order to relieve themselves of the burden of opposing gravity or any other forces at work. In the fully relaxed position, muscular activity stops and the stresses are transferred to the ligaments. The inherent elastic property of the ligaments is sufficient to support most positions with almost nil activity from the surrounding musculature. The ligaments are bearing nearly the entire load, which in the low back consists of the weight of the body above the level concerned. This process is a gradual one, occurring unconsciously over several minutes and varying in time for each individual.

The positions which most commonly stress the low back are the various forms of flexion. When the ligaments are positionally loaded, a constant mechanical stress is being applied to them. In situations of prolonged flexion the posterior ligamentous structures are likely to become elongated and overstretched,[43] which may cause sufficient stress to trigger and fire the nociceptive receptor mechanism. Prolonged stooping, bending and sitting place the low back into prolonged full flexion and are recognised as circumstances which often enhance low back pain. Andersson et al.[9] have described how the myoelectric activity of the back muscles reduces once the ligaments are providing the support in sitting. We can assume safely that this is also the case in prolonged stooping and bending.

It is clear that purely postural or positional mechanisms may produce pain. Thus, frequently low back pain is caused or enhanced by overstretching of ligamentous structures brought about by positions of prolonged flexion. It is my opinion, that all low back pain includes elements of postural stress. Without removing these postural stresses the low back pain patient is doomed to perpetuate his suffering. The importance of the factors, described by Wyke,[4] has not been understood fully by the medical and physiotherapy professions. These factors can nearly all be dealt with by example and education.

Abnormal forces:

Abnormal forces during movement are the cause of most other mechanical back pains. The abnormal forces are most commonly found when heavy loads are manually controlled or when comparatively light weights are handled in great numbers and frequency. Activities involving sudden unexpected movements, such as football, cricket, tennis, athletics, and gymnastics, may sometimes cause enough mechanical stresses to produce low back pain.

A popular misconception

Patients with low back pain commonly complain that their symptoms are worse as a direct result of certain activities. On questioning a patient he will state that his low back has become painful, because he played tennis or football or due to some other activity. He was symptom free prior to and during the exertion, and the *pain commenced following the exertion*. The immediate and generally accepted conclusion is that the activity was in some way harmful to the patient, and the actual exertion has produced significant pain.

When pain is experienced not during but following exertion, it is not often the exertion itself that is responsible for the pain. Mechanical deformation must have occurred in the period following the activity. In the majority of cases the position adopted by the patient while relaxing after activity is responsible for the onset of low back pain. It must be emphasised that *mechanical deformation produced during and as a result of activity will be apparent during the performance of the activity*. The patient may not necessarily feel pain at the time, but usually he will be aware of some damaging sensation.

CHAPTER 4

The Intervertebral Disc

STRUCTURE

In the lumbar spine the intervertebral discs are constructed similarly to those in other parts of the vertebral column. The disc has two distinct components: the annulus fibrosus forming the retaining wall for the nucleus pulposus.

The annulus fibrosus (Fig. 4:1) is constructed of concentric layers of collagen fibres. Each layer lies at an angle to its neighbour and the whole forms a laminated band which holds the two adjacent vertebrae together and retains the nuclear gel. The annulus is attached firmly to the vertebral end plates above and below, except posteriorly where the peripheral attachment of the annulus is not so firm.[14] Moreover, the posterior longitudinal ligament with which the posterior annulus blends is a relatively weak structure, whereas anteriorly the annulus blends intimately with the powerful anterior longitudinal ligament.[14] The posterior part of the annulus is the weakest part: the anterior and lateral portions are approximately twice as thick as the posterior portion, where the layers appear to be narrower and less numerous, the fibres in adjacent layers are oriented more nearly parallel to each other, and there is less binding substance.[17] Due to its structure the annulus fibrosus permits some movement, though small, in all directions.

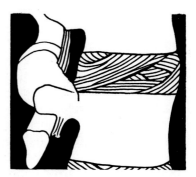

Fig. 4:1.
The annulus fibrosus.

The nucleus pulposus, the central part of the disc, is a transparent jelly, has a high water content, and behaves as a highly viscous fluid.[20] Various authorities[18,19] describe the nucleus as containing as much as eighty-eight percent water at birth, reducing to about seventy-five percent in the third decade and seventy percent in old age.

The size of the disc nucleus and its capacity to swell is greater in the lumbar region than in the cervical or thoracic spine. The capacity to swell when decompressed is evident in the variation in height of man occurring after a nights rest. This diurnal, nocturnal variation is caused by compression forces which reduce mans height during the day as water is squeezed from the disc into the vertebral bodies. The water returns from the vertebral body to the disc with degravitation overnight. Various other authorities have described fluid loss during compressive loading of the discs.[21, 43] Up to five percent of fluid loss is stated to occur during certain compressive movements. Reversal of this flow occurs when the compressive force is removed but Hickey and Hukins state[43] that if movements are performed too rapidly, reversal will not be complete. It is possible then that repetition of a particular movement may cause a progressive loss of fluid resulting in reduced bulk.

The water content of the annulus fibrosus changes less dramatically from seventy-eight percent at birth to seventy percent in middle and old age, so that in ageing the nuclear fluid content reduces to that of the annulus. Perhaps, when the viscosity of nucleus and annulus reaches an equilibrium, internal derangement is less likely to occur. This could account for the decreased incidence of low back pain from age fifty onwards.

Of all the intervertebral discs the lumbar discs are by far the thickest and bear the greatest loading and stresses. Even when slightly degenerated they behave hydrostatically[7] — that is, the pressure within the disc is equally distributed in all directions of the intervertebral compartment.

PRESSURE DISTRIBUTION WITHIN THE DISC

In the young disc the gel structure of the nucleus allows forces, placed on the disc, to be distributed isotropically — that is, evenly around the disc wall. With ageing the soluble content of the nucleus gradually changes into a collagen matrix and the viscosity of the nuclear gel decreases; forces on the disc are now unevenly distributed from nucleus to annulus, probably producing an irregular pattern of comparatively high pressure points at the inner disc wall. In the final stages of disc ageing the nuclear collagen and the inner annular collagen tend to coalesce and the separation between nucleus and annulus becomes ill-defined.[20]

Consequently, where in early life the disc behaves as an ideal shock absorber, in old age the whole system of nucleus and annulus together becomes easily permeable to the fluid in which the collagen is dispersed and the disc tends to behave like a sponge. In middle age, however, the annulus is still separated from the nucleus but contains a matrix of precipitated material, which may distribute compression forces in an uneven manner and could facilitate rupture.[20]

NUCLEAR MOVEMENT

The centre of the lumbar disc nucleus is usually found posterior to the geometric centre of the vertebral body. During movements of the spine a positional change of the nucleus pulposus takes place — for example, from full flexion to full extension there is a small but apparently significant anterior movement of the nucleus of the involved segment. The reverse occurs when the spine moves from extension to flexion. It is this nuclear movement which permits the performance of flexion and extension, and any other movement for that matter.

Many authors have described movements of the nucleus pulposus between the vertebral bodies accompanying alterations in the relative positions of the segments (Fig. 4:2). Armstrong[14] described movement of the nucleus from anterior to posterior occurring during the performance of flexion, and the reverse movement occurring during extension, though he did not have strong laboratory evidence to support his contention. Much later Shah et al[13] demonstrated with discography that the opaque medium injected in the disc moves in a similar way during offset compression loading tests simulating flexion and extension.

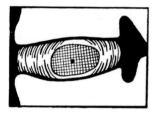 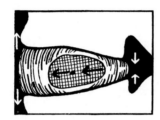 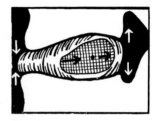

Fig. 4:2a.
The nucleus pulposus with the spine in neutral position.

Fig. 4:2b.
The nucleus pulposus with the spine in extension.

Fig. 4:2c.
The nucleus pulposus with the spine in flexion.

Following laboratory experiments with silastic placed between the vertebral bodies Farfan[21] concluded that evidence acquired this way suggests an ability of the nucleus to move away from the site where compressive forces are applied. The nucleus therefore can in addition to movement in the antero-postero plane move laterally and can inhabit an eccentric position between the vertebral bodies as shown by the discovery of eccentrically placed disc nucleus in the cadavers of people who were known to have had idiopathic scoliosis.[21]

As a result of a continually flexed lifestyle I believe the nucleus may migrate to occupy a more posterior position between the vertebral bodies. (This would account for the approximation of the anterior vertebral margins said to occur in early disc disease.)

TANGENTIAL STRESS

In experiments on lumbar spinal sections of cadavers Shah et al.[13] demonstrated that anterior compression loading of the disc simulating flexion, causes a considerable increase in tangential stress at the posterior annulus, while the anterior annulus bulges. On posterior compression loading simulating extension, the tangential stress reduces posteriorly but increases anteriorly, while the annular bulge disappears anteriorly but appears posteriorly (Fig. 4:3).

It seems that in these situations anterior bulging of the disc wall in flexion and posterior bulging in extension is merely caused by the slack of the relaxed annulus.[43] The bulge is under reduced tangential stress and the nucleus has moved away from the bulge. It is unlikely that nuclear material will be extruded under these circumstances.

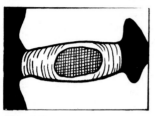 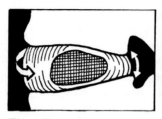 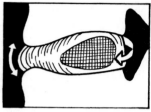

Fig. 4:3a.
Compression loading of the disc.

Fig. 4:3b.
Posterior compression loading of the disc. Tangential stress increased anteriorly — decreased posteriorly. Annulus relaxes posteriorly.

Fig. 4:3c.
Anterior compression loading of the disc. Tangential stress increased posteriorly — decreased anteriorly. Annulus relaxes anteriorly.

I have come to conclude that, *with an intact annular wall, a bulge appearing in the posterior annulus on extension* is normal. In extension the posterior annulus is not under tangential stress and, with the hydrostatic mechanism intact, the nucleus must move anteriorly. It is unlikely that annular tearing will occur under these circumstances.

A bulge appearing in the posterior wall on flexion when the annular wall is damaged may be a threat, as it indicates a weakening posterior annulus. This time the bulge is under increased tangential stress and the nucleus has moved posteriorly. Radial fissuring may occur and nuclear material may occupy this space thus further distending the annulus (Fig. 4:4a).

Fig. 4:4. *Development of disc protrusion.*

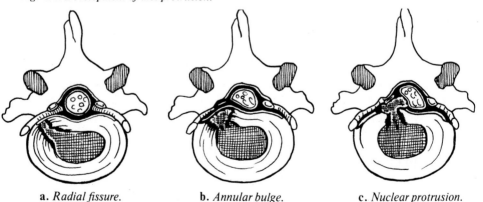

a. *Radial fissure.*   **b.** *Annular bulge.*   **c.** *Nuclear protrusion.*

DISC DAMAGE AND REPAIR

The evidence suggesting that in the lumbar spine the intervertebral disc is a common source of back pain is overwhelming[7, 14, 22, 24, 25] The most convincing signs are the gross kyphosis and scoliosis accompanying severe sciatica. Following laminectomy the patients deformity and sciatica are usually significantly improved. The inference that a disturbance within the disc is responsible for these signs is inescapable. And it is likely that patients who show similar signs but who do not have sciatica, have a similar though lesser disturbance within the disc.

The cause of damage to the disc is still uncertain but it seems unlikely that compression is a significant factor.[14,43] Tension however is considered by various authorities to be a significant factor in the production of damaging stresses especially those affecting the posterior annulus. Brown and co-workers applied a small constant axial load and a repetitive forward bending motion of five degrees and the lumbar discs showed signs of failure after only 200 cycles of bending and completely failed after 1000 cycles. Hickey and Hukins[43] found that bending is particularly damaging because it concentrates stress on a limited number of collagen fibres and if overstretching exceeds four percent irreversible damage occurs.

Markolf[47] describes the spine as being twenty-five to thirty percent less stiff in the flexed position and it can be properly assumed that in this position it is less able to withstand stress.

From my own clinical observations I conclude that the lumbar disc is most commonly damaged in flexed positions especially where flexion is sustained. This usually gives rise to symmetrically distributed pain patterns. Should any torsion or asymetrical stress be applied in addition, the symptoms tend to appear asymetrically. This is manifest by the patients description clinically of the pain first appearing in the back near the mid line and moving laterally and peripherally with the subsequent imposition of torsion.

From the reviewed literature it would appear reasonable to assume that following sustained and repeated flexion stresses the nucleus is forced posteriorly. This coincides with a raising of the intradiscal pressure and increased tangential stress on the postero-lateral disc wall. This happens to be the weakest part of the annular wall, because in this area the annulus has the least radius, is thinner and is least firmly attached to the bone.[14, 17, 23] Should the flexed position be maintained, stress will eventually fatigue the posterior annulus and overcome its inherent strength and should overstretching exceed four percent irreversible damage will result.[43]

The raised intradiscal pressure against the now damaged annulus coupled with the posterior movement of nuclear fluids forces these fluids through the lattice of the weakened collagen and the fibres begin to part. The widening fissure permits nuclear gel to enter the tear accelerating damage and causing separation at the end plate. Should the process continue a significant posterior accumulation of nuclear gel occurs as more and more nucleus is forced down the fissure and eventually bulging occurs at the outer annulus (Fig. 4:4b). Should the tearing be centrally situated the patient exhibits a kyphotic deformity and if the tear extends then posterolaterally the patient will exhibit a scoliotic deformity. When the annular wall is sufficiently weakened by fissuring, extrusion of nuclear material may occur (Fig. 4:4c). The disc has now lost its hydrostatic mechanism and on attempting extension the nucleus is unable to move anteriorly. The ability to extend is seriously impaired, for any approximation of the posterior vertebral rims results in increased pressure on the extrusion itself. This explains why patients with an accomplished protrusion often present with a flattened lumbar spine, and any attempt to extend the low back results in enhancement of low back pain and sciatica.

Farfan[26] has stated that a disc protrusion commences with a tear in the annulus, starting off at the bony vertebral end plate. Tearing must extend to a certacn degree before fragmentation occurs, allowing the annulus to give way. This is nearly always associated with the development of a radial tear which permits the nucleus to force an increase in annular bulging or a widening of the fissure.

Once the disc is damaged by this type of derangement, the natural healing processes will be initiated. Through exposure at the vertebral end plate the vascular tissue of the vertebral body comes in contact with the avascular disc, invading it and removing all the tissue that does not have a blood supply. Scar tissue is now laid down in the inner annulus and nucleus.[26]

Contraction of the invading scar results in the formation of an inelastic structure within the elastic disc. In this way dysfunction develops, causing a loss of mobility in the segment involved. When sufficient stress is applied to the lumbar spine, the scarred areas tend to fragment and tear and the cycle repeats itself.

If we are to prevent the development of dysfunction in the disc following derangement or protrusion, we must provide early movement in our treatment to ensure the formation of an extensible scar within the elastic structure of the disc.

THE DISC AND PAIN

Although the disc does not contain actual nerve endings, it may cause pain in various ways. Severe midline backache may be caused by direct mechanical irritation of the nerve endings in the posterior longitudinal ligament and fibro-adipose tissue, binding the ligament to the annulus. Similarly, pain in or close to the midline of the back may be caused by pressure on the anterior dura mater or its sleeve-like extensions in the intervertebral foramen. These situations occur in central posterior and postero-lateral protrusions of the nucleus pulposus[4] (Fig. 4:5).

Regarding postero-lateral herniation of the nucleus pulposus of a lumbar intervertebral disc Wyke[4] has stated:

"As such a protrusion develops it impinges initially on the sinuvertebral nerve, in which it not only interrupts mechano-receptor afferent activity but may also irritate the contained nociceptive afferent fibres and thereby give rise to pain in the lower back in the absence of sciatica. Should the protrusion develop further, it begins to impinge on the related dorsal nerve roots (and their containing dural sleeves), as a result of which the backache becomes more severe and more widely distributed, and to it are added sensory changes (paraesthesiae and numbness) and pain experienced in the distribution of the sciatic nerve" (Fig. 4:6).

Fig. 4:5. (below)
Posterior or postero-lateral herniation of the nucleus pulposus.

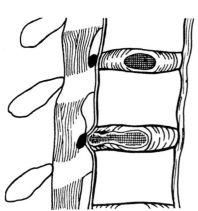

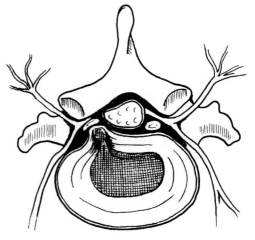

Fig. 4:6. *Postero-lateral herniation of the nucleus pulposus with nerve root compression.*

It can be clearly seen that as this type of lesion develops and worsens, initially the pain is felt in the midline of the back. It progressively increases in intensity and spreads across the back into the buttock and thigh, and as the climax is reached the pain appears in the lower limb. The further from the midline the pain is felt, the greater is the derangement (Fig. 4:7).

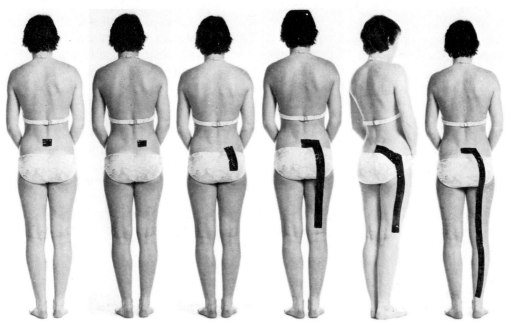

Fig. 4:7. *Pain pattern of a developing lower lumbar disc lesion. When the centralisation phenomenon occurs a reversal of this pattern will be observed.*

THE CENTRALISATION PHENOMENON

In 1959 I noticed in a retrospective observation of case histories that patients who responded rapidly to treatment experienced a centralisation of pain as improvement took place. I called this the 'centralisation phenomenon'.

I would define this phenomenon as the situation in which pain arising from the spine and felt laterally from the midline or distally, is reduced and transferred to a more central or near midline position when certain movements are performed. It is permissable for pain to *increase centrally* provided there is a *reduction* in the *lateral* or *distal* pain.

Centralisation of symptoms only occurs in the derangement syndrome. The significance of the centralisation phenomenon is that in derangement the movement which causes centralisation will, if repeated, reduce the derangement. The phenomenon is not applicable to the dysfunction syndrome and, of course, will not occur in patients with postural problems.

I believe that the centralisation phenomenon is merely the reversal of the development of pain in progressive disc lesions which is described by various authors.[4, 24] As the sequence of symptoms from onset is perfectly logical, so is the reversal of symptoms during centralisation. When the protrusion reduces in size, it releases first the nerve root and then the dura mater, which results in a cessation of pain and paraesthesiae below the knee followed by a reduction in thigh pain. At this stage the pain should be felt mainly in the buttock or central lumbar area.

The typical pattern of pain produced by a developing lower lumbar disc lesion is generally acknowledged. However, it is not always recognised that centralisation as recovery takes place applies to derangement situations and is an indication that reduction of derangement is occurring. Pain of a radiating or referred nature will reduce distally and may simultaneously increase proximally, when the involved joints are moved in the correct direction — that is, reducing the derangement. Thus the pain appears to reverse the order in which it commenced.

The centralisation phenomenon can also be observed in unilateral or symmetrical pain felt solely in the spine. In this case the pain moves from across the low back to a central midline location, and on further reduction of the derangement pain is replaced by an aching or merely a stiffness in the center of the back.

The phenomenon occurs when appropriate movements are performed in the cervical and thoracic spine in the presence of derangement, and is just as reliable.

DIFFERENTIATION BETWEEN
DISC DEGENERATION AND FRANK PROTRUSION

Part [27] has made some observations by discography which have an important clinical implication. He states:

"When there is difficulty in differentiating disc degeneration with annulus rupture from frank nuclear protrusion, flexion and extension films can be helpful. In disc degeneration, forward flexion opens the posterior disc widely, the annulus fibrosus and posterior longitudinal ligament become tightly stretched and the contrast medium tends to disperse uniformly. This is a helpful indication of the true state of affairs in those patients where the contrast appears localised in the neutral or extended positions. On the other hand, when frank nuclear prolapse is present, the opaque medium remains contained in a localised area irrespective of the position of the spine."

The assessment of the effects of certain chosen movements — the test movements — on the pain will enable us to make a clinical diagnosis. In frank nuclear protrusion the hydrostatic mechanism of the disc is impaired, and the position of the nucleus cannot be influenced by movement and positioning. Clinically, the patient's symptoms will not reduce as a result of the test movements, and such a patient is not likely to benefit from mechanical treatment utilising movements and position.

On the other hand, where the disc merely shows degeneration with annular fissuring and no protrusion exists, the hydrostatic mechanism is still intact and the position or shape of the nucleus can be influenced by movement and positioning. Clinically, there will be a change in intensity or site of the patient's symptoms as a result of the test movements, and such a patient can be treated successfully with mechanical procedures utilising movement and positioning.

If disturbance of the normal intervertebral disc mechanism is a causative factor in low back pain it conveniently explains the behaviour of pain, movement and deformity found in patients with the derangement syndrome.

In the postural syndrome, by my definition, no pathology will be found.

In the dysfunction syndrome pathology affecting muscles, ligaments, disc, apophyseal joints and fascias may be found separately or together.

CHAPTER 5

Diagnosis

THE THERAPIST'S RESPONSIBILITY

The therapist is part of the team involved in the treatment and rehabilitation of patients suffering low back pain. In some countries manipulative therapists are primary contact practitioners. Consequently, their diagnostic skills have greatly improved, enabling them to define which mechanical conditions can be helped by mechanical therapy and to separate these conditions from the non-mechanical lesions which have no place in the therapy clinic.

However, differential diagnosis is really not within the scope of manipulative therapy. It is my view that differential diagnosing by medical practitioners is necessary to exclude serious and unsuitable pathologies from being referred for mechanical therapy. In making diagnoses the manipulative therapist should confine himself to musculo-skeletal mechanical lesions. Specialised in this field, he is usually able to make far more accurate diagnoses than most medical practitioners. As the manipulative therapy profession gains international respect, we may soon see the day that this specialisation becomes generally accepted.

DIAGNOSTIC DIFFICULTIES

In the low back mechanical diagnosis is extremely difficult. As yet, no means have been devised which enable us to selectively stress individual structures and identify the source of many pains. As Nachemson[7] states, there is only one condition which allows a fairly confident diagnosis to be made:

> "the patient with sciatica caused by sequestration from the disc which impinges on a nerve root. Such patients, though, represent only a small proportion of those who have low back pain problems, and constitute at most only a few percent."

This means that perhaps as many as ninety percent of patients cannot be diagnosed in a very specific manner. Various authorities[28, 29] have stated that in many instances it is impossible to define the exact pathological basis for low back pain and, consequently, to achieve a precise diagnosis. Nachemson has said:[30]

> "No one in the world knows the real cause of back pain and I am no exception."

When authorities such as these clearly state that the problems surrounding specific diagnosis of low back pain are insurmountable, it seems that the time has come to alter the rules of the game. Instead of aiming for a specific diagnosis based on a particular pathology, we must apply an alternative system of assessment. This can be used until further development of our knowledge and diagnostic procedures enables us to become more specific.

In order to analyse mechanical low back pain and categorise the symptoms a new approach is necessary. I believe we have a means of overcoming the present diagnostic impasse. If mechanical pain is caused by mechanical deformation of soft tissues containing nociceptive receptors, we must confine our diagnosis within this framework.

THE THREE SYNDROMES

All spinal pain of mechanical origin can be classified in one of the following syndromes:

The postural syndrome:

This is caused by mechanical deformation of soft tissues as a result of postural stresses. Maintenance of certain postures or positions which place some soft tissues under prolonged stress, will eventually be productive of pain. Thus, the postural syndrome is characterised by intermittent pain brought on by particular postures or positions, and usually some time must pass before the pain becomes apparent. The pain ceases only with a change of position or after postural correction.

The dysfunction syndrome:

This is caused by mechanical deformation of soft tissues affected by adaptive shortening. Adaptive shortening may occur for a variety of reasons which will be discussed later. It leads to a loss of movement in certain directions and causes pain to be produced before normal full range of movement is achieved. Thus, the dysfunction syndrome is characterised by intermittent pain and a partial loss of movement. The pain is brought on as soon as shortened structures are stressed by end positioning or end movement and ceases almost immediately when the stress is released.

The derangement syndrome:

This is caused by mechanical deformation of soft tissues as a result of internal derangement. Alteration of the position of the fluid nucleus within the disc, and possibly the surrounding annulus, causes a disturbance in the normal resting position of the two vertebrae enclosing the disc involved. Various forms and degrees of internal derangement are possible, and each presents a somewhat different set of signs and symptoms. These will be discussed later. Thus, the derangement syndrome is usually characterised by constant pain, but intermittent pain may occur depending on the size and location of the derangement. There is a partial loss of movement, some movements being full range and others partially or completely blocked. This causes the deformities in kyphosis and scoliosis so typical of the syndrome in the acute stage.

The three syndromes presented are totally different from each other, and each syndrome must be treated as an entity on its own, requiring special procedures which are often unsuitable for the other syndromes. In order to identify which syndrome is present in a particular patient a history must be established and an examination must be performed. The method of history taking and examination is discussed in the following chapters.

CHAPTER 6

The History

Taking an accurate history is the most important part of the initial consultation when one is dealing with any medical or surgical problem. Unfortunately, when the mechanical lesion is involved there is still lack of understanding regarding the nature of the questions that should be asked, the reasons for asking them, and the conclusions to be drawn from the answers.

I will set out step by step the stages that should be developed in history taking, and the questions that should be asked at each stage. Practitioners will already have their own method of history taking, and I do not suggest at all that they should alter their routine. However, I believe that the following questions *must* be included, if one is to reach a conclusion following the examination of patients with mechanical low back pain.

INTERROGATION

As well as the usual questions regarding name, age and address, one should enquire as to the occupation of the patient, in particular his *position at work* which provides us with the most important and relevant information. Managers are not always sitting down as we tend to believe, and postmen are not always walking.

Where is the present pain being felt?

We need to know all the details about the location of the pain, because this will give us some indication of the level and extent of the lesion and the severity of the condition. If there are any associated symptoms such as anaesthesia, paraesthesiae and numbness, their location must be noted as well. Referred pain indicates that derangement is likely.

Because the location of the pain can change rapidly and dramatically, we must find out if the pain has been present on the same site or sites since the onset.

At this stage we must determine whether the symptoms are central, bilateral or unilateral in origin, as this is an important factor in the classification of the patient and consequently in his treatment. Bilateral symptoms indicate a central origin, whereas central symptoms cannot arise from a unilateral structure.[24]

How long has the pain been present?

It is important to find out whether we are dealing with an acute, a subacute or chronic condition. In recurrent low back pain we are not interested in an answer based on the length of time since the *first* attack; at this stage of the examination we want to know how long the *present* episode has been evident.

If the symptoms have been present for any length of time, as is often the case, we must find out whether the patient feels that his condition is improving, stationary or worsening.

The length of time that the condition has been present may assist us to determine the stability of healing following a disc prolapse. It may also indicate the development of dysfunction which is likely to occur following trauma or derangement. The longer the symptoms have been present, the greater are the chances that adaptive changes have taken place.

The length of time that the patient has had symptoms can also guide us in deciding how vigorous we can be with our examining procedures. If a patient has had his symptoms for several months and has been able to work all this time, he will probably have placed more stress on the joints at fault than we are likely to do during the examination, which means that we can be fairly vigorous. If on the other hand the patient had a sudden onset of pain within the past two weeks, we could be dealing with a derangement situation and may well increase the degree of derangement with out test procedures which, if applied too vigorously, may significantly worsen the condition of the patient. Generally speaking, if the condition has been present only for a few days to two or three weeks, we must take great care in handling and exercising the patient; but if the present pain has been evident for months, we can be rather vigorous with our procedures.

How did the pain commence?

Basically we want to find out if there was an apparent or no apparent reason for the onset of the pain. Most of the histories commonly state that the pain appeared for no apparent reason. Two of every three patients fall into this category, and only one patient will recognise a causative strain.

If pain has arisen for an apparent reason a recognisable strain has caused the symptoms — for example, an accident, a sports injury, lifting. If the patient was involved in an accident — for example, if he were struck by a bus, — he may have sustained multiple injuries and the mechanics of none of these would be clear. This type of patient must be treated gently and with caution.

If pain has arisen for no apparent reason, a derangement or dysfunction has developed during the course of normal living usually without the application of any external force. Strains arising in this fashion can under most circumstances be avoided by modification of the patient's daily living habits or movements. However, if the pain commenced for no apparent reason and is gradually and insidiously worsening, we may well suspect serious pathology, particularly if the patient feels or looks unwell at the time of interrogation. It is always better to suspect the worst and be wrong, than to overlook the worst and be wrong.

Careful evaluation of the patient's information regarding the onset of his symptoms is necessary in order to avoid faulty conclusions. There are situations in which the patient thinks that his pain commenced for no apparent reason, whereas we may recognise a causative strain; alternatively the patient may wrongfully relate the onset to certain activities in an attempt to find a cause for his low back pain, which in fact appeared for quite different reasons.

Is the pain constant or intermittent?

This is the most important question we must ask patients with low back pain. If in patients referred for mechanical therapy the pain is found to be constant, it usually is produced by constant mechanical deformation. However, we must keep in mind that constant pain can also be caused by chemical irritation. Intermittent pain is always produced by mechanical deformation.

Constant chemical pain:

This is present as long as chemical irritants are present in sufficient quantities and occurs in inflammatory and infective disorders and in the first ten to twenty days following trauma. Chemical pain following trauma reduces steadily as healing takes place. Chemical irritants do not appear and disappear during the course of the day. Therefore, pain of chemical origin is always constant, and patients who describe periods in the day when no pain is present must have intermittent pain which is of mechanical and not of chemical origin.

Mechanical stresses that would normally be painless, can become painful where chemical irritation has raised the threshold of excitation of the nociceptive receptors. Thus, *movements may superimpose mechanical forces on an existing chemical pain and enhance it, but they will never reduce or abolish chemical pain*. This is significant in the differentiation between chemical and mechanical pain.

Low back pain caused by chemical irritation is comparatively easy to identify, as the pain is usually constant and no mechanical means can be found to significantly reduce it. Five days of treatment and observation should be sufficient to arrive at this conclusion.

Constant and intermittent mechanical pain:

This is present as long as mechanical stresses are sufficient to cause mechanical deformation. This type of pain will frequently reduce or even disappear when movements or positions are adopted that sufficiently reduce the mechanical stresses. On the other hand, the mechanical stresses may as easily be increased by movements and positions. *Constant mechanical pain will vary significantly in intensity but never disappears, whereas intermittent mechanical pain appears and disappears according to circumstances.*

Constant pain must be truly constant — that is, there is *no time in the day when pain or aching is not present*. Pain must be classified as intermittent even if there is only half an hour in the day when the patient feels completely painfree. In that half hour there is no mechanical deformation present, and we must examine the circumstances in which the patient is painfree and utilise this information for treatment purposes. It is much simpler to treat a patient who has intermittent pain than one whose pain is constant and in whom mechanical deformation is present under all circumstances.

It is my observation that about seventy percent of low back pain patients have intermittent pain, and the remaining thirty percent have truly constant pain. The majority of patients with constant mechanical pain are likely to belong to the derangement category. Derangement alters the tension in the structures about the segment involved, increasing mechanical deformation in some tissues and decreasing it in others. The constant increase in tension produces constant pain which continues, until the tension is decreased by reduction of the derangement or adaptive lengthening of surrounding tissues.

Intermittent pain is relatively easy to treat, because if there is one hour in the day when no mechanical deformation is present, it is possible to gradually extend that painfree time period. Constant pain is rather a different problem and is more difficult to treat. The percentage of patients failing to respond to treatment is higher in the constant pain group than in the intermittent pain group. Generally speaking, the derangement syndrome can be associated with constant pain, whereas the postural and dysfunctional syndromes are characterised by intermittent pain.

What makes the pain worse? and What makes the pain better?

We must specifically ask about sitting, standing, walking, lying, and activities which involve stooping or prolonged stooping. In these positions the joint mechanics of the lumbar spine are relatively well understood, and therefore we will be able to determine which situations increase and which decrease mechanical deformation. We must carefully record any position or activity reported to reduce or relieve the pain, as we will utilise this information in our initial treatment.

Sitting:

In relaxed or prolonged sitting the lumbar spine falls into full flexion, the effects of which are described in detail elsewhere (Chapter 2). If a patient tells us that sitting increases his symptoms, we know that sustained flexion causes mechanical deformation of his lumbar spine. But if a patient finds relief in sitting, flexion actually reduces the mechanical deformation.

Standing:

Standing, expecially relaxed standing, places the lower lumbar spine in full end range extension which means that certain structures are on full stretch. If a patient tells us that he is worse in relaxed standing, sustained maximum extension produces mechanical deformation of his lower lumbar spine. But if a patient finds relief in relaxed standing, sustained maximum extension reduces the mechanical deformation.

Walking:

Walking accentuates extension — that is, it further increases the lordosis of the lumbar spine as the hind leg by its backward movement brings the pelvis into forward inclination. If walking produces or increases pain, extension must produce or increase mechanical deformation of the lower lumbar spine. But if the patient has no pain in walking, extension is reducing the mechanical deformation.

Lying:

There are basically three positions which may be adopted while lying: prone, supine and side lying. The many variations of these, caused by different leg positions, make evaluation of the effects of lying rather difficult. Apart from the lying position itself, the effects on the lumbar spine depend on the nature of the surface on which one lies — usually the mattress and its supporting base — which may be firm and unyielding, or soft and giving.

The effects of the three basic positions on the lumbar spine can be summarised as follows:

(a) In *lying supine* on a firm surface the lumbar spine falls into extension, whereas on a soft surface the degree of extension is decreased and in some cases flexion may be produced.

(b) In *lying prone* on a firm as well as a soft surface the lumbar spine is always placed near or at full end range of extension.

(c) In *side lying* the lumbar spine is brought into side gliding towards the side one is lying on, more so when on a soft surface than on a hard surface.

Activities which involve bending:

In bending or prolonged bending the lumbar spine falls into full flexion and added to this are gravitational stresses. If, for example, gardening produces pain, sustained flexion must produce mechanical deformation of the lumbar spine. But if the pain is reduced while gardening, sustained flexion stops the mechanical deformation.

Patients who have had pain for a long time, may have difficulty in determining what makes their pain better or worse. They are no longer able to observe objectively their own pain patterns because of the length of time the pain has been present. It is necessary to spend extra time to extract detailed information regarding the pain behaviour, because without this we cannot proceed to an adequate conclusion and appropriate treatment.

Occasionally a patient will tell us that there is no position or movement which affects the pain. In this case the information obtained from the history is insufficient, and during the examination we must try to produce a change in the patient's symptoms by utilising extremes of movement or sustained positions.

Have there been previous episodes of low back pain?

We should enquire about the nature of any similar or other low back pain episodes, the time span over which they occurred, and their frequency. At this stage we should also find out about previous treatments and their results. Episodic history indicates derangement. Dysfunction is likely to develop insidiously after each episode and will now coexist but be masked by the present disturbance. Its presence will be revealed after resolution of pain resulting from the derangement.

Further questions

> pain on cough/sneeze?
> disturbed sleep?
> pain on arising in the morning?
> recent X-Rays? — results?
> on medication at present?
> on steroids, in past or at present?
> general health? — recent weight loss?
> major surgery or accident, recently or previously?
> saddle anaesthesia? — bladder control?

Information gained from these questions may complete the picture of the condition we are dealing with. The reasons for asking these questions are obvious and straight forward, and they will not be discussed in detail.

Although the referring medical practitioner will almost certainly have excluded any serious or unsuitable pathology, we must remain alert for its presence.

Fig. 6:1. (opposite.) *Lumbar spine assessment sheet.*

LUMBAR SPINE ASSESSMENT

Date ....

Name ....

Address ....

....

Date of birth ....

Occupation ....

HISTORY

Symptoms now ....

....

at onset ....

Present for ....

Commenced as a result of ....

No apparent reason. ☐

Constant/Intermittent.

When worse —   bending,   sitting or rising from,   standing,   walking,   lying.

Other ....

When better —   bending,   sitting or rising from,   standing,   walking,   lying.

Other ....

Disturbed sleep — Yes   No   Cough/sneeze +ve —ve

Previous history ....

and treatment ....

X-Rays ....

General health ....   Meds/Steroids ....

Recent surgery ....   Accident ....

Gait ....   Bladder ....

EXAMINATION

Posture sitting ....   Lordosis reduced/accentuated ....

Posture standing ....   Leg length ....

Lateral shift (R) or (L) or nil

....

MOVEMENT LOSS

Flexion: Major.   Moderate.   Minimal.   Deviation (R) or (L) ....

Extension: Major.   Moderate.   Minimal.   Deviation (R) or (L) ....

Side Gliding: (R) or (L) ....

TEST MOVEMENTS

FIS ....   SGIS (R) ....

REP. FIS ....   SGIS (L) ....

EIS ....   REP. SGIS (R) ....

REP. EIS ....   REP. SGIS (L) ....

FIL ....

REP. FIL ....

EIL ....

REP. EIL ....

Neurological ....

Hip joints ....   S.I.

Conclusion: Posture   Dysfunction   Derangement

PRINCIPLE OF TREATMENT

The Examination

Having digested the information supplied by the referring doctor, extracted as much relevant information as possible from the patient, and checked the radiologist's report, we may proceed to the examination proper.

If the patient is able to do so, we should make him sit on a straight backed chair while taking his history. During this time he will reveal the true nature of his sitting posture. When the patient rises to undress after the interrogation we should observe the way he rises from sitting, his gait, the way he moves, and any deformity that may be obvious.

We will record the following:

I. POSTURE SITTING

If the patient has been sitting during history taking, we already have a good impression of his posture (Fig. 7:1). We now ask him to sit on the edge of the examination table with his back unsupported. In the majority of cases the patient will sit slouched with a flexed lumbar spine. Some patients are more aware of the relationship between their posture and pain. They have discovered that they can control their sitting pain by sitting upright and may sit very well on first observation. Unfortunately, these patients are few and far between.

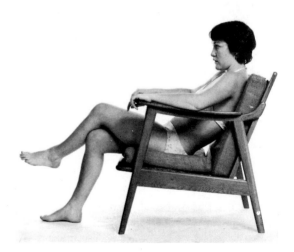

Fig. 7:1.
Relaxed sitting posture.

II. POSTURE STANDING

We examine in particular the following features:

1. Reduced or accentuated lordosis

The most common postural fault to be observed in the standing position is the flattened lumbar spine or reduced lordosis (Fig. 7:2a). Some patients have a deformity in kyphosis.

Another common deformity or departure from the 'norm' is the patient exhibiting an accentuated lumbar lordosis (Fig. 7:2b). Though much less common than the flattened spine this is clearly a separate category and should be treated accordingly.

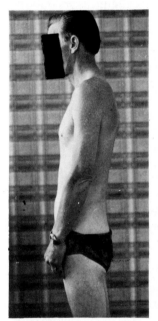 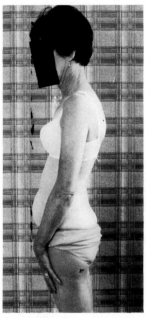 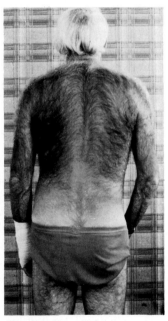

Fig. 7:2a.
Reduced lumbar lordosis.

Fig. 7:2b.
Accentuated lumbar lordosis.

Fig. 7:2c.
Lateral shift to the right.

2. Lateral shift

A departure from the midline causing a lumbar scoliosis or lateral shift is evident in about fifty-two percent of patients.[10] There are many reasons for the lumbar spine to depart even slightly from the midline: the anatomical configuration of the joint surfaces may dictate this; a congenital anomaly may be present; there may be some remote mechanical cause; and an alteration in the position of the disc nucleus may be responsible.

The lateral shift is sometimes barely discernable, and great care must be taken to ensure that the deformity is not overlooked (Fig. 7:2c). This is important because some movements, especially extension, produce pain when performed in the presence of a lateral shift, whereas if there was no shift they would be painfree. We must never fail to recognise a minor lateral shift and its possible role in the production of symptoms.

I have chosen to describe a right lateral shift — or a lateral shift to the right — as the situation which exists, when the vetebra above has rotated and laterally flexed to the right in relation to the vertebra below, carrying the trunk with it. Thus the top half of the patient's body has moved to his right in relation to the bottom half.

3. Leg length discrepancy

If a leg length discrepancy is encountered, we must investigate the relevance of the discrepancy to the patient's symptoms. When in the history there is no record of pain being enhanced by standing and walking, the difference in leg length is not likely to be relevant. But when pain is produced by standing or walking, we should increase the length of the short leg to bring about symmetry and await the effect of this on the patient's symptoms. When relevant, leg length adjustment causes a fairly rapid change in the symptoms experienced during standing and walking. This change should become apparent within a few days at the most.

There are various methods of measuring the leg length, but the only truly reliable way to detect minor differences in leg lengths is by taking an x-ray of the pelvis and both full legs with the patient in standing. However, it is doubtful that minor leg length discrepancies cause significant low back pain.

At this stage, with the patient still standing, it may be advisable to quickly test the integrity of the conduction of the lower lumbar and upper sacral nerve roots. Therefore we ask the patient to walk on his toes and then on his heels. In case of difficulty or when in doubt about the outcome a more detailed neurological examination must be performed.

III. EXAMINATION OF MOVEMENT

Here we are interested in observing the quality of the movement itself — that is, the range of movement and the movement pathway. We will determine if there is a movement loss and if deviation from the normal movement path takes place. The word 'pain' should not be mentioned until we are ready to assess the effects of the movements on pain.

The patient should be standing with his feet about thirty centimeters apart and only one movement will be performed in the direction to be evaluated. We examine:

1. Flexion

This is the first movement to be examined, because in patients with dysfunction or derangement the flexion movement provides us with the most relevant information regarding the nature and the degree of the disturbance. The standing patient is asked to run the hands down the front of both legs, moving as far as possible into flexed standing, followed immediately by returning to neutral standing (Fig. 7:3).

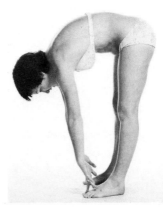

Fig. 7:3.
Examination of movement — flexion.

Any loss of flexion should be noted. Loss of flexion manifests itself in one of two ways: either the end range of flexion is limited, or a deviation from the normal pathway of flexion has developed. In some patients with a severe loss of flexion end range, the lumbar lordosis is still present after the patient has bent forward as far as possible, in others the lumbar spine merely remains flat. Any asymmetrical impediment to flexion may cause the spine to take the path of least resistance, resulting in a deviation from the sagittal pathway. By far the majority of patients with a flexion loss divert from the sagittal plane during flexion and deviate to one side or the other of the midline. This may occur in an arc-type of movement, the flexion commencing and ending in midline positions; or, once movement is commenced, it may divert from the midline and increase its departure for as long as flexion is continued.

Deviation in Flexion

In my experience there are three clearly defined and separate causes for deviation in flexion. The mechanism is different in each case and the treatment must be varied accordingly. Thus deviation in flexion may be due to:

(a) Derangement within the vertebral joint. In this situation the altered position of the fluid nucleus compels a deviant flexion pathway. Generally, the deviation in flexion occurs away from the painful side as long as there is no sciatic nerve root irritation. In some patients the deviation is variable and will occur one day to the left and the next day to the right.

(b) Dysfunction within the vertebral joint. This develops following repair of damage after derangement. In this situation the consequent scarring by fibrous connective tissue prevents flexion in the sagittal plane and the deviation may take place towards or away from the painful side, but is never variable.

(c) Dysfunction external to the vertebral joint. This exists in the presence of an entrapped or adherent sciatic nerve root. In this situation the root is no longer able to lengthen adequately and allow flexion to occur in the sagittal plane. It will now act as an anchor and pull the patient during flexion towards the side of root adherence. The *deviation in flexion may become very severe and always take place towards the painful side.*

2. Extension

The standing patient is asked to place his hands in the small of the back and bend backwards as far as possible, followed immediately by returning to neutral standing (Fig. 7:4).

The loss of some degree of extension is very common after the age of thirty. Any limitation of extension evident in the lumbar spine should be recorded as well as the presence of a deviation in the extension pathway which is occasionally encountered. Major disc bulging will cause a deviation in extension away from the side of the pain and enhancement of sciatica will occur. However, facet apposition in full extension usually prevents significant deviation.

3. Side gliding

Having considered over the past twenty-five years the relevance of the information obtained by assessing the movements of rotation and side bending separately, I have come to the conclusion that it is better to combine the two movements in the one movement of side gliding.

In order to examine side gliding the standing patient is asked to move his shoulders and pelvis simultaneously in opposite directions while keeping the shoulders parallel to the ground. As some patients have difficulty in performing this movement, it may be necessary to assist the patient by guiding the movement with a hand placed on one of his shoulders and the other hand on his oppositic iliac crest (Fig. 7:5).

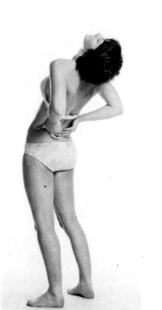
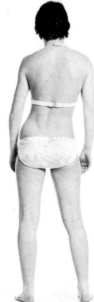

Fig. 7:4 (right)
Examination of movement —
extension.

Fig. 7:5. (far right)
Examination of movement —
side gliding.

The side gliding movement is frequently unilaterally impaired. When the patient has a lateral shift, there is always some unilateral loss of side gliding. In this situation the movement is restricted or completely blocked in the direction opposite to the lateral shift.

IV. MOVEMENTS IN RELATION TO PAIN

After examining the lumbar spine in relation to function, we must now investigate the effects of various movements on the pain. Let us assume that pain is produced by mechanical deformation as described by Wyke.[4] As discussed before, stresses applied to soft tissues will under certain circumstances be productive of pain. Any attempt to *force normal movement* (application of abnormal stress) in a joint with a visibly *impaired function* (abnormal tissue), must result in the production or enhancement of pain.

In order to stress the joints in a controlled manner and avoid exacerbation I have devised a sequence of test movements, the mechanics of which are relatively well understood and the effects of which can be controlled. By applying the test movements during the examination we will enhance pain under some circumstances and reduce it in others. Information gained by deliberately stressing the joints is vital and enables us to select and categorise patients into three groups — that is, patients with pain arising from postural, dysfunctional or derangemental causes.

The test movements are first performed in standing and then in lying. When performed in lying they must be done in such a way that the effect on the lumbar spine is a passive stretch, and any form of active movement produced by the muscles surrounding the lumbar spine should be avoided. In this way we can achieve a better end range stress than with active movements.

When the *test movements are performed in standing* a normal stress is applied to normal or abnormal tissue; in the former case no pain will be produced; in the latter case pain will be produced or increased if the test movements enhance the mechanical deformation, but pain will be decreased or abolished if the test movements reduce the mechanical deformation. When the *test movements are performed in lying* a passive stress is added by the patient and an abnormal stress is applied to normal or abnormal tissue; in the former case no pain should result, because the stress is not excessive and is only applied momentarily; in the latter case pain will be produced or increased if the test movements enhance the mechanical deformation, but pain will be decreased or abolished if the test movements reduce the mechanical deformation.

If we are to relate movements to pain, the test movements must be performed in such a way that they produce a change in the patient's symptoms. This change may be brought about in various ways: if prior to movement pain is present, the test movement may increase or reduce its intensity; it may alter the site of the pain by centralisation or by abolishing one pain and introducing another one. If prior to movement no pain is present, the test movement may produce the pain complained of.

If there is no change in the patient's symptoms during or immediately following the test movements, the joints have not been stressed adequately and the process should be repeated more vigorously. It may also be that the pain is not of mechanical origin, because mechanical pain *must be* and *always is* affected by movement or position. Or, alternatively, the lumbar spine is not causing the problems and other areas should be investigated.

REPEATED MOVEMENTS

When assessing the results of the test movements it is important to examine the effects of repeating them. Repeated movements are vital in the examination of spinal segments when disc pathology is suspected and it is necessary to determine if a derangement situation exists. It is my belief that with movement of the vertebral column the nucleus can alter its shape, and with sustained positions or repeated movements it will eventually alter its position. Clinically this manifests itself in the derangement syndrome by a change in intensity or site of the symptoms. A decrease or centralisation of pain is absolutely reliable in indicating which movement should be chosen to reduce mechanical deformation. I have learnt to rely implicitly on centralisation as the most important clinical guide to establish the correct direction of movement which will reduce derangement. An increase or peripheralisation of pain is just as reliable in indicating which movement should be avoided because it enhances mechanical deformation. If there is an increase or peripheralisation of pain when performing any technique or movement, a worsening of the condition of the patient is likely. There is one exception to this rule: the patient with an adherent nerve root in chronic sciatica. There are special tests which easily identify this condition, and these will be discussed later.

In derangement the performance of repeated movements in the direction which increases accumulation of nuclear material will result in a progressively increasing derangement and increasing or peripheralising pain. The performance of repeated movements in the opposite direction will result in a reduction of the derangement and reduction or centralisation of pain. Thus, repeated movements are diagnostic in derangement pathologies.

In dysfunction the performance of repeated movements in the direction which stretches adaptively shortened structures will produce pain at the end range of movement, but repetition does not make the patient progressively worse. When he returns to the neutral position the pain will disappear. Thus, repeated movements are diagnostic in dysfunction as well.

Patients with the postural syndrome will not experience pain with any of the test movements or their repetition. These patients must be positioned in order to have their pain reproduced.

Apart from exposing the derangement and dysfunction syndromes, repeated movements are essential in determining whether the timing is appropriate to commence stretching procedures following trauma and derangement. *When repeated movements, applied to painful structures, produce less and less pain with each repetition these structures should be exercised.* On the other hand, *when more and more pain is experienced with each repetition exercising is not indicated* and more time should be allowed for the condition to heal. *This fundamental response of pain sensitive structures to stress must be applied to soft tissue lesions throughout the musculo-skeletal system in order to determine whether a passive or an active treatment approach should be developed.*

The movements that I have chosen as test movements are the ones of flexion, extension and side gliding. In my experience these movements will induce or reduce mechanical deformation in the lumbar spine quicker and more effectively than any other movement. Generally speaking, the movements that produce the greatest amount of mechanical deformation and therefore pain can, when reversed or modified, be used to have the greatest effect on the reduction of that mechanical deformation and pain. For example, rotation is rarely complained of as producing significant pain and therefore neither enhances nor reduces mechanical deformation significantly. On the other hand, flexion and extension are commonly stated to be the most painful movements and are potentially the most useful movements for treatment purposes.

Different effects are produced when the tests movements are performed in standing compared with lying. This requires further discussion for both flexion and extension.

Flexion in standing compared with flexion in lying

In the test movements flexion of the lumbar spine is examined in two ways: in standing by bending the trunk forwards; and in supine lying by using the hands to passively bend the knees onto the chest. Apart from the obvious difference achieved by removal of gravitational stress in flexion in lying, there are two major points to note:

In flexion in lying the flexion takes place from below upwards, the L5-S1 joint moving first followed by flexion in turn of each successively higher segment. On the other hand, in flexion in standing the flexion occurs from above downwards.

A better flexion stretch is obtained, especially at L5-S1, by the passively performed flexion in lying, and patients with flexion dysfunction describe a stretch pain in flexion in lying which they may not experience in flexion in standing. Frequently in flexion in lying, pain is produced immediately when the movement commences and the pain increases as the degree of flexion increases. Thus, in flexion in lying pain is produced as soon as the L5-S1 segment (and perhaps L4-L5) is placed under full stretch which occurs immediately flexion is initiated. In flexion in standing the pain will only be experienced at the end of the movement, because only when flexion in standing is almost full are the L4-L5-S1 segments stretched to the full.

The effects on the sciatic nerve roots are different in flexion in standing and flexion in lying. In flexion in standing the sciatic nerve is fully lengthened and placed on full stretch, producing effects identical to those obtained in straight-leg-raising tests. Flexion in lying, when performed with simultaneous hip and knee flexion as described, has no such effect and root adherance or root tension can not be identified in this manner.

The production or enhancement of sciatic pain by flexion in standing may be caused by a bulging disc or an adherent root. However, production or enhancement of sciatic pain by flexion in lying can only be caused by a bulging disc. We have now at our disposal a simple test to differentiate between disc bulging and root adherence. No one should persist with the performance of flexion in lying in the presence of *increasing* referred pain. Such perserverance can be rewarded by the production of a severe disc lesion.

Extension in standing compared with extension in lying

In the test movements extension of the lumbar spine is examined in two ways: in standing by bending the trunk backwards; and in prone lying by passively raising the trunk, using the arms instead of the back muscles and at the same time keeping the pelvis down. Both manoeuvres cause extension of the lumbar spine from above downwards. There are two major points to note:

The gravitational forces applied to the joints are different in extension in lying and extension in standing. In extension in lying the weight of pelvis and abdomen causes an increase of extension range in the joints of the low back. The force exerted is almost perpendicular to the plane of the body and has a maximal mechanical effect. In extension in standing the gravitational forces act on the joints of the low back at an angle of up to forty five degrees from perpendicular and are therefore less efficient. The greatest extension stretch that a person can apply to his own back is by performing extension in lying. The extension range and stretch are never as complete in extension in standing.

In extension in standing the compressive forces appear sometimes sufficient to prevent full end range movement. This would indicate that some derangements are too large to be reduced in the presence of compressive forces in standing. However, reduction of the same derangements becomes possible in the prone lying position, when the vertical compressive forces are removed.

I believe that there must be other factors, unexplained as yet, which contribute to the purely mechanical effects of exercises performed in lying and in standing. Gravitational or compressive forces alone do not account for the nature of the differences which can be observed clinically.

THE TEST MOVEMENTS

All patients should perform the test movements except when they are in such severe pain that it is intolerable to do so. This only occurs in major derangement situations, and it may be necessary to place such patients on bed rest in order to facilitate reduction of the derangement by removing gravitational stresses. After a period of twenty-four to forty-eight hours in bed, positioned so that reduction may be enhanced, re-assessment should follow.

Flexion in standing

The patient, standing with his feet about thirty centimeters apart, is asked to run his hands down the front of both legs as far as range and pain allow (Fig. 7:6). He then immediately returns to neutral standing. With the hands actually placed on the legs the more acute or insecure patients will feel safer in performing flexion. Flexion in standing is performed once and its effects on the pain are recorded. The movement should then be repeated up to ten times and the effects of repetition recorded. We must ensure that maximum possible stretch is obtained during the last few movements.

For example: Flexion in standing — produces (R) buttock pain at end range.
Repeated flexion in standing — worsens (R) buttock pain and produces (R) calf pain.

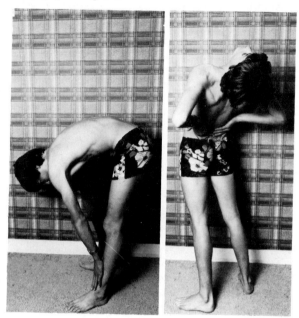

Fig. 7:6. (right)
Test movements — flexion in standing.

Fig. 7:7. (far right)
Test movements — extension in standing.

Extension in standing

The patient, standing with the hands in the small of the back to act as a fulcrum, is asked to bend backwards as far as possible (Fig. 7:7). He then immediately returns to netural standing. The test movement is performed once and its effects on the pain are recorded. The movement should then be repeated up to ten times and the effects of repetition recorded. We must ensure that maximum possible stretch is obtained during the last few movements.

For example: Extension in standing — produces central back pain.
Repeated extenstion in standing — reduces central back pain.

If extension in standing increases or peripheralises the pain, we must consider the possibility of the presence of a lateral shift. If a lateral shift is present and is relevant to the patient's symptoms, the performance of any of the test movements with the shift uncorrected will always increase mechanical deformation and thus enhance pain. Extension in standing following shift correction will reduce the derangement and thus decrease the pain.

Side gliding in standing

This is done to determine whether side gliding increases or decreases mechanical deformation and, in the presence of a lateral shift, to test the relevance of the shift to the patient's symptoms.

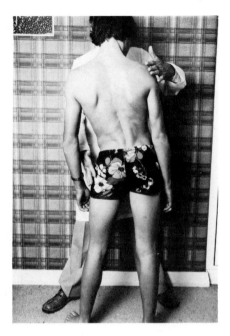

Fig. 7:8.
Test movements — side gliding in standing with operator-assistance.

As some patients find it difficult to perform side gliding in standing the examiner may initially have to assist this movement. The patient stands in front of the examiner, who places one hand on one of the patient's shoulders and the other hand on the patient's opposite iliac crest. The examiner presses both hands towards the midline, causing a major movement of the top half of the patient's body in relation to the bottom half (Fig. 7:8). Instead of applying the pressure on the patient's shoulder, it may under certain circumstances be preferable to press against the side of his rib cage. In all instances both shoulders of the patient should remain parallel to the ground. Side gliding must be tested first in the one and then in the other direction, before the sequence is repeated. The effects of the test movements on the pain should be recorded.

> For example: (L) side gliding — increases (R) buttock pain and produces (R) calf pain.
> (R) side gliding — reduced (R) buttock and calf pain.
> Repeated (L) side gliding — not indicated as it is likely to worsen the symptoms.
> Repeated (R) side gliding — reduces (R) buttock pain, abolishes (R) calf pain.

When side gliding is found to be painful and blocked usually a lateral shift is present and in the treatment therapist assistance may be required.

When side gliding is found to be painful but not blocked, a lateral shift is unlikely to be present and in the treatment, therapist assistance is usually unnecessary.

When assessing the relevance of a lateral shift, we must determine whether the shift results from the same mechanical distrubance which has produced the patient's pain. The shift is considered to be relevant when the movement of side gliding alters the site or intensity of the pain. If no pain change occurs during the performance of side gliding to the one side or the other, the scoliosis cannot be considered part of the mechanical problem causing pain.

Flexion in lying

The patient, lying supine with the knees flexed and the feet flat on the couch, is asked to bend the knees onto the chest. Clasping the knees with his hands he applies a firm pressure to produce maximum possible lumbar flexion (Fig. 7:9). The legs are then lowered to the starting position. The effects of the first test movement on the pain are recorded. The movement should then be repeated up to ten times, ensuring that the maximum possible stretch is obtained during the last few movements. The effects of repetition are recorded.

For example: Flexion in lying — increases pain (R) L5.
                     Repeated flexion in lying — worsens pain (R) L5 and produces (R) buttock pain.

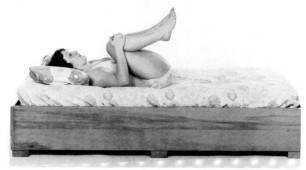

Fig. 7:9.
Test movements — flexion in lying.

Extension in lying

The patient, lying prone with the hands directly under the shoulders as in the traditional press-up position, is asked to raise the top half of his body by straightening the arms, at the same time keeping the thighs and legs on the couch (Fig. 7:10). If the pelvis lifts from the couch as the arms are straightened, we must make sure that the low back is allowed to sag as much as possible. The patient then returns to the starting position. The effects of this movement on the pain are recorded. The movement should then be repeated up to ten times, ensuring that the maximum possible stretch is obtained during the last few movements. Again, the effects of repetition are recorded.

For example: Extension in lying — reduces (L) buttock pain.
                Repeated extension in lying — abolishes (L) buttock pain and produces central low back pain.

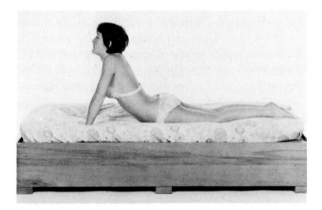

Fig. 7:10.
Test movements — extension in lying.

The test movements should be performed in a certain sequence. The examiner should not deviate from this method, unless it is obvious that to persist will inflict unnecessary pain on the patient.

In abbreviated form the sequence of test movements is as follows:

FIS	(flexion in standing)
Rep FIS	(repeated flexion in standing)
EIS	(extension in standing)
Rep EIS	(repeated extension in standing)
SGIS	(right and left side gliding in standing)
Rep SGIS	(repeated right and left side gliding in standing)
FIL	(flexion in lying)
Rep FIL	(repeated flexion in lying)
EIL	(extension in lying)
Rep EIL	(repeated extension in lying)

V. OTHER EXAMINATION PROCEDURES

At this stage it is appropriate to test the mobility of the hip joints and the integrity of the sacro-iliac joints, if these are thought to contribute to the problems of the patient. Should passive stretching of the various structures about the hip reproduce the symptoms complained of, this joint must be considered a possible source of the pain. The sacro-iliac joints, although not commonly the cause of low back pain, turn out to be involved often enough to make a fool of those failing to check them. In my opinion the tests described by Cyriax[31] are adequate to determine if the symptoms are arising from these joints. (Testing of sacro-iliac structures by using bony prominences as land marks and attributing pain to asymmetries so located is dishonest.)

A more detailed neurological examination may be required, if there is the slightest suggestion of nerve root or spinal cord signs. In these cases the patient's symptoms will be felt in the lower limb. Further neurological examination should include testing of reflexes, muscle strength and sensation.

VI. CONCLUSIONS

The correlation of information from history, examination and test movements will indicate whether the patient is suffering from the postural, derangemental or dysfunctional syndrome. This differentiation is essential, as it indicates which principle of treatment should be used.

Postural correction

In the postural syndrome postural correction is the only treatment required.

The extension principle

In posterior derangement the extension principle should be applied when *extension reduces* mechanical deformation. Thus in the treatment we are making use of those movements which *centralised, decreased or stopped the pain* during the examination. The patient should receive mechanical therapy based on the principle of extension. This includes: passive extension, extension mobilisation, extension manipulation, extension in standing, extension in lying, and sustained extension.

Patients with an acute lumbar scoliosis or a lateral shift are placed in the extension principle category once correction of the lateral deformity has been achieved.

In dysfunction, however, the extension principle should be applied when *extension produces* mechanical deformation. Thus in the treatment we are making use of those movements which actually *produced the pain* during the examination. For treatment of dysfunction to be successful it is imperative that some pain be experienced, especially in the initial stages when adaptively shortened tissues must be stretched enough to assist them to regain their original length and elasticity. Pain thus produced during treatment of extension dysfunction must always be across the back and near the midline, and significant buttock pain should not occur. The treatment procedures are based on the principle of extension (see above).

The flexion principle

In anterior derangement the flexion principle should be applied when *flexion reduces* mechanical deformation. Again, in the treatment we are making use of those movements which *centralised, decreased or stopped the pain* during the examination. The treatment consists of procedures based on the principle of flexion. This includes: flexion mobilisation, flexion manipulation, flexion in lying, and flexion in standing.

In dysfunction, however, the flexion principle should be applied when *flexion produces* mechanical deformation, and in the treatment we use those movements which actually *produced the pain* during the examination. Some pain must be experienced in treatment of flexion dysfunction to be effective and treatment consists of procedures utilising flexion (see above).

Generally speaking:

in the treatment of derangement we must choose the movement that relieves the pain, as this movement decreases the mechanical deformation by reducing the derangement.

but:

in the treatment of dysfunction we must always choose the movement that produces the pain, as this movement will gradually stretch and lengthen contracted soft tissues, eventually reducing mechanical deformation.

About seventy-five to eighty percent of all the patients with low back pain will respond to the extension and flexion programmes. These patients have a very good chance of becoming independent of therapists. They will be able to perform exercises to relieve themselves of pain without requiring techniques performed by specialist therapists. The remaining twenty to twenty-five percent of patients will require special techniques and manipulative procedures. The experienced practitioner will be able to identify these patients with a trial of test procedures carried out over a twenty-four hour period.

Hopefully at this stage we will be able to categorise patients into the appropriate syndrome and adopt a principle of treatment. We are now ready to teach the patient how to correct the posture, restore lost function and, where possible, reduce derangement himself.

I will proceed with a discussion of the procedures which may be used in treatment, as these will be frequently referred to in chapters to follow. Then I will consider the three syndromes and their respective treatment approaches individually.

CHAPTER 8

Technique

There are many differing philosophies and concepts surrounding the practise of spinal manipulation and its effects on the pathologies which may exist in the spine. To satisfy all these philosophies an equal number of institutions has developed, teaching those wishing to learn. No matter what school presents its case or which philosophy is adhered to, all manipulative specialists claim to have a high success rate. They all use techniques which vary in nature, application and intent; they proclaim that their own methods are superior to those used by others; and yet, somehow they all obtain uniformly good results. Self-limitation of low back pain plays, of course, a significant role in this happy situation. Apart from this there are definite benefits which are obtained quickly by using manipulative techniques.

Throughout the years I have practised many forms of mobilisation and manipulation, including osteopathic and chiropractic techniques and those taught by Cyriax. I have come to believe that it is immaterial which manipulative school or philosophy one upholds for, no matter what particular manipulations are used, the results of technique appear to be the same. The general procedures of Cyriax are just as effective as the finely developed specific procedures of the osteopaths and chiropractors.

It is now well documented[32, 33] that asymmetries in the facet joints and other developmental anomalies occur as regularly in the lumbar region as in the other areas of the spine, and are present in up to fifty-two percent of the population. Where palpable movement restrictions and departures from the typical exist, it is impossible to state that these are either the cause of the patient's present symptoms or are likely to cause symptoms in the future. To conclude that palpable anomalies should be mobilised is no longer a tenable suggestion. One may well be dealing with perfectly 'normal' and asymptomatic asymmetrical lumbar articulations.

Diagnosis by palpation is relevent only when associated with the increase and decrease of mechanical deformation. Those who claim to 'feel' restrictions by palpation and simultaneously fail to reproduce the patient's symptoms, are only fooling themselves and their patients. Enthusiasts searching for sacro-iliac pathology are frequently misled by this philosophy. The production of pain at a certain level by palpation and passive movement is not enough to justify treatment at that level. The pain produced *must* be the one that has forced consultation — not a new pain induced by the palpation.

49

Various manipulative authorities maintain that mobilisation or manipulation of a hypermobile spinal segment should be avoided at all times. This is excellent advice when it applies to pathological hypermobilities as fractures and spondylolisthesis. However, a hypermobile joint in itself is considered by some to cause mechanical pain more readily than joints with a normal or decreased mobility. I must emphasise that a hypermobile joint becomes painful in the same manner as any other joint. When it is placed on full stretch for a long enough period or when the stretch is severe enough pain will be felt. It so happens that in the hypermobile segment a greater range of movement must be accomplished before full stretch is achieved. Thus, hypermobility is not in itself a painful state.

The basic misunderstanding that passive movements applied to a hypermobile joint are harmful, has led to the systematic development of techniques of specific manipulation which spare the hypermobile joints and affect only the adjacent hypomobile joints. It has also brought about unjustified condemnation of those who advocate general instead of specific manipulation.

Many people have criticised and rejected the techniques of Cyriax which are considered to be unselective, non-specific and rather coarse in their application. However, at this time hundreds of Cyriax-trained doctors and physiotherapists successfully apply his methods in many parts of the world and it appears that no harm is caused by his approach. If general manipulation were damaging indeed, then by now there would be enough evidence to support this contention. I am sure that the antagonists of Cyriax would not have allowed any compromising situation to pass unnoticed.

Unfortunately, it appears that some manipulative schools attempt to enhance the quality and mystique of their skills by increasing the complexity of their techniques. They create the impression that to master the art and science of manipulation one must acquire very complex skills; these are possessed and taught only by an elite group, and if one wishes to enjoy the highest reputation in manipulation one must join this elite group; the only way to do this is to train at an exclusive establishment. This continuing trend is a threat to the scientific development of mechanical therapy.

The procedures which I have chosen for the treatment of low back pain are totally unsophisticated and non-specific. In general, the techniques affect many segments and localisation is not attempted. However, these procedures have an *immediate cause and effect* on the patient's symptoms. The reasons put forth for their effectiveness may prove to be wrong in the future, but the effectiveness itself will not change: if patients are selected as suggested and the techniques are applied as suggested, the procedures will be as effective fifty years from now as they are today.

It is one of the main theses of this book that patients can be taught to manage, treat and control their own low back pain. In order to achieve this it is necessary to depart from the traditional methods of mechanical treatment, whereby the therapist *does something to* the patient to bring about change. In that case the patient attributes his recovery, rightly or wrongly, to what was *done to* him and for all future episodes of low back pain he commits himself to the care of the therapist. By avoiding the use of therapist-technique in the initial stages of treatment and substituting patient-technique, the patient will recognise that his recovery is clearly the result of his own efforts. Only few patients fail to assume responsibility for active participation in their treatment.

At present a great deal of research and academic discussion is taking place in attempts to establish the scientific validation of manipulation and explain its effects.[34] The most obvious and most important effect of mobilisation and manipulation is the increase of range of movement at any joint to which the techniques are applied. This may be caused by a change in the position of an internal structure, or by such an alteration in an adjacent structure that a more normal function is possible than existed prior to the application of the technique. The increase in range of movement as obtained by manipulation and mobilisation can also be achieved by exercises when performed in a certain way.

It is my belief that an exercise becomes a mobilisation when performed with a certain frequency and in such a way that a rhythmical passive stretch is created. And in a similar manner a passive mobilisation can become a manipulation. The suggestion put forth is that mobilisation and manipulation are nothing more than extended exercises, and an exercise can therefore become a mobilisation or manipulation. Therapy based on self-mobilisation and self-manipulation has arrived and *it is possible to teach patients to practise mobilisation and manipulation of their own spine.*

Provided there is adequate instruction and careful explanation regarding the aims of treatment, the self-treatment concept can be applied successfully to most low back pain patients — that is, to all the patients with the postural syndrome, nearly all with the dysfunction syndrome, and about seventy-five percent of the patients with the derangement syndrome. Thus, twenty-five to thirty percent of patients with low back pain will not recover on the exercise programme alone, and need additional techniques of either mobilisation or manipulation which must be applied by a specialist therapist. The only equipment required to treat patients is an adjustable treatment table, the height of which can be varied and which has an end section of about two feet that can be inclined up or down.

THE PROCEDURES AND THEIR EFFECTS

After much investigation to determine the optimum number of movements necessary to effect stretching of shortened tissues and alteration in the position of the fluid nucleus, I have come to conclude that usually any significant change will occur within ten to fifteen repetitions of the procedure and no benefit will be obtained by exceeding this number. Therefore, exercises are performed in series of ten to fifteen excursions each. The number of times in the day that a series of exercises must be done varies according to the syndrome to be treated, the effects to be obtained, and the capabilities of the patient involved.

Unless stated otherwise, exercises will be performed with an almost continuous rhythm. On each contraction the maximum possible range must be maintained for a second or two. Each excursion *must* be followed by relaxation, and a brief pause of only a fraction of a second is required. Normally patients can complete between ten to fifteen excursions in one minute. Therefore no patient should use the excuse that he has not got enough time to do the exercises as instructed.

In assessing progress the evaluation of pain changes is vital. A patient can improve in several ways: the intensity of the pain may reduce; the frequency with which the pain occurs may decrease; or the site of the pain may alter. Centralisation of the pain indicates that the patient is improving, although in terms of intensity he may still feel one hundred percent of the pain originally complained of. In this case an explanation of the pain behaviour usually satisfies the patient regarding his progress.

If the site of pain has not changed on the patient's next visit, I always enquire about the frequency and intensity of the pain in the following manner: "If you had one hundred units of pain on your last visit, how many do you have today in terms of (a) frequency; and (b) intensity?".

The procedures include patient-technique as well as therapist-technique. In order to facilitate quick reference the procedures are summarised below.

TABLE OF PROCEDURES

Procedure 1 : lying prone

2 : lying prone in extension

3 : extension in lying

4 : extension in lying with belt fixation

5 : sustained extension

6 : extension in standing

7 : extension mobilisation

8 : extension manipulation

9 : rotation mobilisation in extension

10 : rotation manipulation in extension

11 : sustained rotation/mobilisation in flexion

12 : rotation manipulation in flexion

13 : flexion in lying

14 : flexion in standing

15 : flexion in step standing

16 : correction of lateral shift

17 : self-correction of lateral shift

PROCEDURE 1 — LYING PRONE

The patient adopts the prone lying position with the arms alongside the trunk and the head turned to one side. In this position the lumbar spine falls automatically into some degree of lordosis (Fig. 8:1).

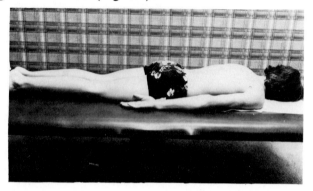

Fig. 8:1.
Lying prone.

Effects:

In derangement with some degree of posterior displacement of the nuclear content of the disc the adoption of procedure 1 may cause, or contribute to, the reduction of the derangement provided enough time is allowed for the fluid nucleus to alter its position anteriorly. A period of five to ten minutes of relaxed prone lying is usually sufficient. This procedure is essential and the first step to be taken in the treatment and self-treatment of derangement.

In patients with *a major derangement,* such as those presenting with an acute lumbar kyphosis, the natural lordosis of prone lying is unobtainable. These patients cannot tolerate the prone position unless they are lying over a few pillows, supporting their deformity in kyphosis.

In minor derangement situations the degree of posterior movement of the nucleus is relatively small. Prone lying may actually reduce the derangement without any other procedures being required in the treatment, provided sufficient time is allowed for the fluid mechanism to alter to a more anterior position. In these situations the prone position, though obtainable, may initially be painful. This does not indicate that the procedure is undesirable. The increase of pain in this position is nearly always felt centrally and is in fact desirable. If pain is produced or enhanced peripherally, the prone position must be considered harmful and should not be maintained.

A basic requirement for the self-treatment of derangement is that the prone position can be obtained and maintained. In this position the patient will commence the self-manipulative procedures, based on the extension principle.

In dysfunction there is a loss of extension movement or a reduced lordosis. In some patients with extension dysfunction the loss of movement may be enough to prevent lying prone for more than a few minutes. For these people lying prone in bed or while sunbathing has become impossible, because soft tissue shortening has reduced the available range of movement and prolonged extension stress produces pain.

The prone lying procedure by itself is not sufficient to resolve extension dysfunction. However, when adopted regularly and in conjunction with other procedures, prone lying should become painless as lengthening of shortened tissues takes place.

The prone lying position should be obtained by all patients attending for treatment of low back pain. It has been suggested that this position can be harmful because it increases and accentuates the lumbar lordosis. This applies only in a few situations: when we have failed to correct a relevant lateral shift prior to assuming the prone lying position; when extension produces or increases the compression on the sciatic nerve root; and in those rare derangements where nuclear material has accumulated anteriorly or antero-laterally, and prone lying increases the derangement. In all other instances the prone lying position is highly beneficial.

Patients with posterior derangement should after reduction be careful when arising from the prone position to standing. Every effort must be made to maintain the restored lordosis while moving from lying to standing in order to maintain the reduction of the derangement.

PROCEDURE 2 — LYING PRONE IN EXTENSION

The patient, already lying prone, places the elbows under the shoulders and raises the top half of his body so that he comes to lean on elbows and forearms while pelvis and thighs remain on the couch. In this position the lumbar lordosis is automatically increased. Emphasis must be placed on allowing the low back to sag and the lordosis to increase (Fig. 8:2).

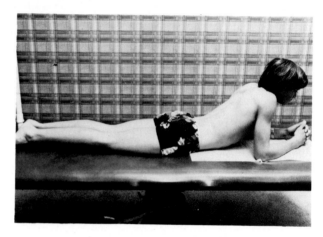

Fig. 8:2.
Lying prone in extension.

Effects:

Procedure 2 is a progression of procedure 1 and merely enhances its effects by increasing extension.

Again, in derangement some time must be allowed to affect the contents of the disc and, if possible patients should remain in this position for five to ten minutes. In more acute patients sustained extension may not be well tolerated due to pain, and initially we must rely on the use of intermittent extension.

PROCEDURE 3 — EXTENSION IN LYING

The patient, already lying prone, places the hands (palms down) near the shoulders as for the traditional press-up exercise. He now presses the top half of his body up by straightening the arms, while the bottom half, from the pelvis down is allowed to sag with gravity. The top half of the body is then lowered and the exercise is repeated about ten times. The first two or three movements should be carried out with some caution, but once these are found to be safe the remaining extension stresses may become successively stronger until the last movement is made to the *maximum possible extension range*. If the first series of exercises appears beneficial, then a second series may be indicated. More vigour can be applied and a better effect will be obtained if the last two or three extension stresses are sustained for a few seconds.

It is essential to obtain the maximum elevation by the tenth excursion and once obtained the lumbar spine should be permitted to relax into the most extreme 'sagged' position (Fig. 8:3).

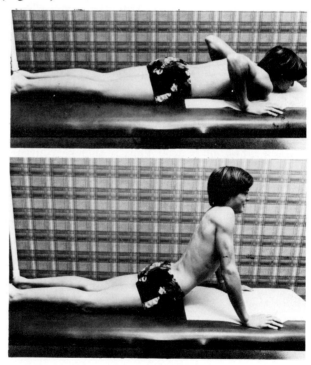

Fig. 8:3.
Extension in lying.

Effects:

This procedure is a further progression of the previous two. Instead of a sustained extension stress on the contents and surrounding structures of the lumbar segments, there is now an intermittent extension stress, having a pumping as well as a stretching effect.

This procedure is the most important and effective in the treatment of derangement as well as extension dysfunction. The very maximum degree of extension possible without external assistance, is obtained with this exercise. An increase of central low back pain at maximum elevation can be expected and should not cause any concern as it will gradually wear off. It is usually described as a strain pain and differs from the pain which has caused initial consultation.

In addition to the effects on the disc and periarticular structures there are two other physiologically related phenomena that could possibly result from the performance of this exercise.

The self sealing phenomenon

Evidence gathered by Markolf and Morris[46] suggests that a self sealing mechanism exists within the disc and appears shortly after injury. The initial injury weakens the annulus but appropriate stress applied subsequently results in restoration of near normal strength, suggesting that the disc has a remarkable recovery ability and that certain stresses may enhance rapid recovery. White and Panjabi[44] conclude that the self sealing phenomena is mechanical in nature and is not dependent on the viscosity or softness of the disc, for the study was performed on degenerative as well as normal discs.

My question arising from this information is . . . Does the performance of repeated passive extension in lying cause a reversal of the posterior migration of the nucleus into the developing radial fissure? Does the movement then initiate the self sealing phenomena?

Cartilaginous repair

Following trauma articular surfaces are normally rested or immobilised to permit healing. It is well known that scar tissue is laid down under these circumstances and damaged articular cartilage is replaced with fibrous collagen. Recent investigations by Salter[48] suggest that if passive continuous motion is applied to joints containing traumatised intra articular cartilage, the damaged cartilage is replaced by true cartilaginous cells instead of scar tissue, and further, these joints do not develop arthritic changes subsequently. The evidence has yet to be confirmed in human studies. We can now pose the question . . . Does the regular performance of passive extension following lumbar disc damage enhance the quality or improve the nature of the healing tissues of the posterior annulus?

PROCEDURE 4 — EXTENSION IN LYING WITH BELT FIXATION

The patient's position and the exercise are the same as in the third procedure, but now a fixating belt is placed at or just below the segments to be extended. The safety belt is the first simple external aid, used to enhance maximum extension. It does so by preventing the pelvis and lumbar spine lifting from the couch. Other methods of restraint may be used effectively, for example the body weight of a young son or daughter when exercising at home (Fig. 8:4).

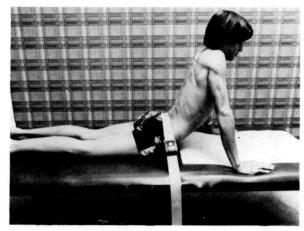

Fig. 8:4.
Extension in lying with belt fixation.

Effects:

This procedure creates a greater and more localised passive extension stress than the previous ones. It is particularly suitable for stretching in the case of extension dysfunction, and is more often required in dysfunction than in derangement.

In dysfunction some pain will be experienced in the small of the back while exercising, because contracted tissues are being stretched. In derangement the rules pertaining to the centralisation phenomenon must be observed, and the procedure stopped if peripheral pain is produced or increased.

PROCEDURE 5 — SUSTAINED EXTENSION

To apply a sustained extension stress to the lumbar spine an adjustable couch, one end of which may be raised, is a necessary piece of equipment. The patient lies prone with his head at the adjustable end of the couch which is gradually raised, about one to two inches at the time over a five to ten minute period. Once the maximum possible degree of extension is reached, the position may be held for two to ten minutes, according to the patient's tolerance. When lowering the patient the adjustable end of the couch should slowly be returned to the horizontal over a period of two to three minutes. This must not be done rapidly, for acute low back pain may result (Fig. 8:5).

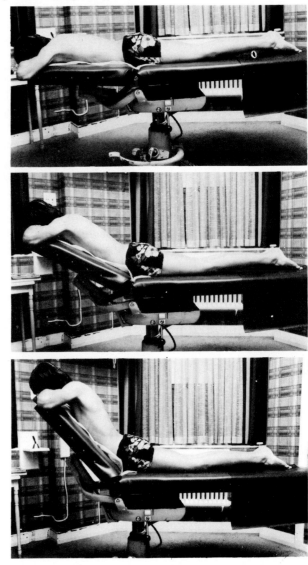

Fig. 8:5.
Sustained extension.

Effects:

The procedure is predominantly used in the treatment of derangement. The effect is similar to that of the third procedure, but a time factor is added with the graduated increase and the sustained nature of the extension. In certain circumstances a sustained extension stress is preferable to a repeated extension stress.

The centralisation phenomenon must be watched closely. Any suggestion that the pain is moving or increasing peripherally must lead to the immediate but *slow* lowering of the couch. It is interesting to note that *an increase in central low back pain as the couch is lowered nearly always indicates a good response to the treatment, whereas when there is no increase in central pain patients tend to have little or no improvement following this procedure.*

PROCEDURE 6 — EXTENSION IN STANDING

The patient stands with the feet well apart and places the hands (fingers pointing backwards) in the small of the back across the belt line. He leans backwards as far as possible, using the hands as a fulcrum, and then returns to neutral standing. The exercise is repeated about ten times. As with extension in lying it is necessary to move to the very maximum to obtain the desired result (Fig. 8:6).

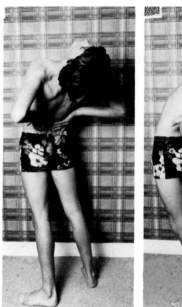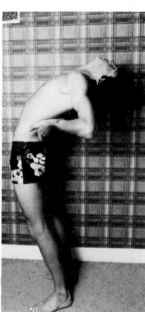

Fig. 8:6.
Extension in standing.

Effects:

Extension in standing produces similar effects on derangement and dysfunction as extension in lying, but it is less effective in the earlier treatment stages of both syndromes. Whenever extension in lying is prevented by circumstances, an extension stress can be given by extension in standing.

In derangement, extension in standing is designed to reduce accumulation of nuclear material in the posterior compartment of the intervertebral joint, provided this accumulation is not gross. In the latter case extension in lying will have to be performed first. The procedure is very important in the *prevention of the onset of low back pain* during or after prolonged sitting or activities involving prolonged stooping, and is *very effective when performed before pain is actually felt.*

PROCEDURE 7 — EXTENSION MOBILISATION

The patient lies prone as for procedure 1. The therapist stands to one side of the patient, crosses the arms and places the heels of the hands on the transverse processes of the appropriate lumbar segment. A gentle pressure is applied symmetrically and immediately released, but the hands must not lose contact. This is repeated rhythmically to the same segment about ten times. Each pressure is a little stronger than the previous one, depending on the patient's tolerance and the behaviour of the pain. The procedure should be applied to the adjacent segments, one at a time, until all the areas affected have been mobilised (Fig. 8:7).

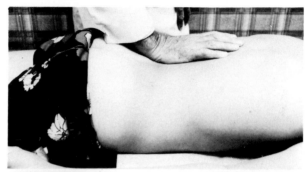

Fig. 8:7a.

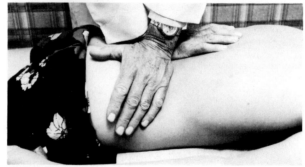

Fig. 8:7b.

Fig. 8:7c.

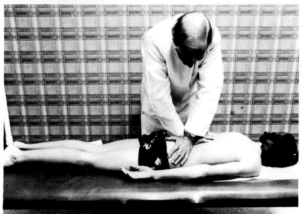

Fig. 8:7a and b.
Positioning of hands prior to extension mobilisation.

Fig. 8:7c.
Extension mobilisation.

Effects:

In this procedure the external force applied by the therapist enhances the effects on derangement and dysfunction as described for the previous extension procedures.

In general, symmetrical pressures are used on patients with central and bilateral symptoms. Therapist-technique must be added when the patient is unable to reduce derangement or resolve dysfunction by the self-treatment procedures. That situation appears in derangement when instead of progressively *lessening* pain extension in lying (procedure 3) causes the *same* pain with each repetition. Under those circumstances extension mobilisation is indicated.

PROCEDURE 8 — EXTENSION MANIPULATION

There are many techniques devised for manipulation of the lumbar spine in extension. It is not important which technique is used, provided the technique is performed on the properly selected patient and applied in the correct direction. The technique that I recommend is similar to the first two manipulations described by Cyriax[31] for the reduction of a lumbar disc lesion.

The patient lies prone as for procedure 1. The therapist stands to one side of the patient and, having selected the affected segment, places the hands on either side of the spine as for the technique of extension mobilisation (procedure 7), which is always applied as a premanipulative testing procedure. If following testing the manipulation is indicated, the therapist leans over the patient with the arms at right angles to the spine and forces slowly downwards until the spine feels taut. Then a high velocity thrust of very short amplitude is applied and immediately released (Fig. 8:8).

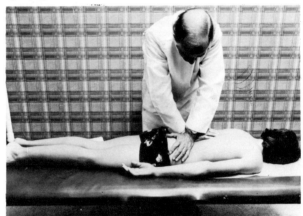

Fig. 8:8.
Extension manipulation.

Effects:

The effects of the external force and the reasons for its use are the same as for procedure 7. When the desired result is not obtained with the mobilising techniques, manipulation is indicated under certain circumstances.

The extension thrust is used by many manipulators, and there is difference of opinion regarding the structures that may be influenced by this technique. Cyriax[31] states that it reduces derangement of an annular fragment of the disc. Others propose reduction of facet locking, tearing of adhesions and reduction of nerve root entrapment. Whatever the true mechanism may be, properly selected patients often experience a click or a dull thud. In most instances the click is followed by a change, usually an improvement, in the patient's signs and symptoms.

PROCEDURE 9 — ROTATION MOBILISATION IN EXTENSION

The position of patient and therapist is the same as for procedure 7. By modifying the technique of extension mobilisation so that the pressure is applied first to the transverse process on the one side and then on the other side of the appropriate segment a rocking effect is obtained. Each time the vertebra is rotated away from the side to which the pressure is applied — for example, pressure on the right transverse process of the fourth lumbar vertebra causes left rotation of the same vertebra. The technique should be repeated about ten times on the involved segment and, if indicated, adjacent segments should be treated as well (Fig. 8:9).

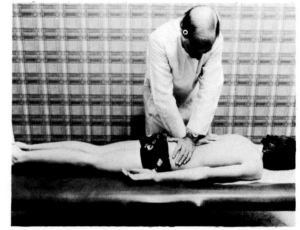

Fig. 8:9.
Rotation mobilisation in extension.

Effects:

Also here the external force applied by the therapist enhances the effects on derangement and dysfunction as described for the previous extension procedures. The reasons for adding therapist-technique are the same as for procedure 7.

In general, unilateral techniques are likely to effect unilateral or asymmetrical symptoms sooner and more efficiently than bilateral or central techniques. But once centralisation of symptoms has taken place, treatment may be continued with central or bilateral techniques. Thus, in derangement rotation mobilisation in extension may have to be performed first to bring about centralisation of nuclear material in the disc. This is followed by symmetrical extension mobilisation to restore the nucleus to its more anterior position.

Occasionally a click is felt during mobilisation. A click often indicates a reduction of derangement, and we should immediately assess if this is the case. If the patient has improved significantly as a result of this technique, any further treatment may disturb the reduction and the treatment session should be terminated at this point.

During the procedure the patient may describe an enhancement of the pain by pressure on one side with a corresponding reduction of the pain by pressure on the other side. This is valuable information on which further treatment will be based. We must keep in mind that we are affecting the pain by increasing or decreasing mechanical deformation. *In dysfunction an increase in mechanical deformation with certain limits is desirable* and pain should be produced or increased with the application of the technique. *In derangement an increase in mechanical deformation is extremely undesirable,* and we should aim for a decrease instead with centralisation, reduction or abolition of the pain. Therefore, precise identification of the syndrome to be treated is essential to determine whether rotation mobilisation should be performed towards the painful or the painfree side.

PROCEDURE 10 — ROTATION MANIPULATION IN EXTENSION

The patient lies prone as for procedure 1. The therapist stands to one side of the patient and, having selected the correct segment, places the hands on either side of the spine as for the technique of rotation mobilisation in extension (procedure 9), which is always applied as a premanipulative testing procedure. The information obtained from the mobilisation is vital and determines on which side and in which direction the manipulation is to be performed. If following testing the manipulation is indicated, the therapist reinforces the one hand with the other on the appropriate transverse process. The manipulation is then performed as in procedure 8 (Fig. 8:10).

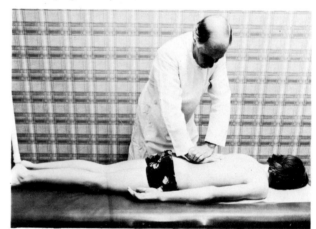

Fig. 8:10.
Rotation manipulation in extension.

Effects:

The effects of the external force and the reasons for its use are the same as for procedure 9. When the desired result is not obtained with the mobilising technique, manipulation is indicated under certain circumstances. Regarding the direction in which the manipulation is to be performed the same rules apply as for procedure 9.

PROCEDURE 11 —
SUSTAINED ROTATION/MOBILISATION IN FLEXION

The patient lies supine on the couch, and the therapist stands on the side to which the legs are to be drawn, facing the head end of the couch. The patient's far shoulder is held firmly on the couch by the therapist's near hand, providing fixation and stabilisation. With the other hand the therapist flexes the patient's hips and knees to a rightangle and carries them towards himself, causing the lumbar spine to rotate. With the patient's ankles resting on the therapist's thigh the knees are allowed to sink as far as possible and the legs are permitted to rest in that extreme position. The lumbar spine is now hanging on its ligaments in a position which combines side bending and rotation. By pushing the knees further towards the floor the therapist applies overpressure to take up the remaining slack in the lumbar spine. Depending on the purpose for which the procedure is used, the position of extreme rotation is maintained for a shorter or longer period (Fig. 8:11).

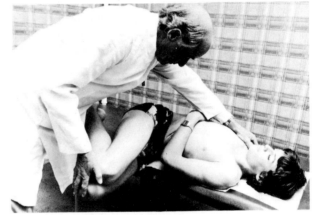

Fig. 8:11.
Sustained rotation/mobilisation in flexion.

Effects:

The procedure is mainly used in derangement. Sustained rotation for about thirty to forty seconds provides the time factor required to allow alteration of the position of the fluid nucleus within the disc. In those situations where time is important in the reduction this procedure may effect relief that will not be obtained by the much quicker performed rotation thrust (procedure 12). During the period that rotation is sustained the patient should be watched closely and asked constantly about the behaviour of pain. Any sign of peripheralisation of symptoms indicates that more than enough time has been spent in this position.

The procedure may also be used as a mobilising technique in dysfunction, or as premanipulative testing in dysfunction as well as in derangement. In these cases the rotation is less sustained or performed in a rhythmical mobilising manner.

If a small therapist cannot reach across the patient to stabilise his shoulder, a seat belt fastened firmly across the patient's upper chest provides adequate fixation. Alternatively, a second person may be used to hold the patient down.

The Lumbar Spine

PROCEDURE 12 — ROTATION MANIPULATION IN FLEXION

The sequence of procedure 11 must be followed completely to perform the required pre-manipulative testing. If the manipulation is indicated a sudden thrust of high velocity and small amplitude is performed, moving the spine into extreme side bending and rotation (Fig. 8:12).

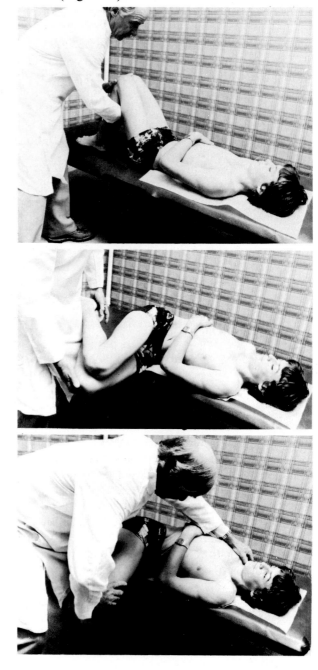

Fig. 8:12.
Rotation manipulation in flexion.

Effects:

There are many techniques devised for rotation manipulation of the lumbar spine. When rotation of the lumbar spine is achieved by using the legs of the patient as a lever or fulcrum of movement, confusion arises as to the direction in which the lumbar spine rotates. This is judged by the movement of the upper vertebrae in relation to the lower — for example, if the patient is lying supine and the legs are taken to the right, then the lumbar spine rotates to the left.

It has become widely accepted that rotation manipulation of the spine should be performed by rotation away from the painful side. This has applied to derangement as well as dysfunction, because hitherto no differentiation has been made between these syndromes. I wish to emphasise that, while this practise is correct for the majority of derangements, it is useless at best when applied to dysfunction. Because there are more low back pain patients with dysfunction than with derangement, it is essential to determine precisely which syndrome is present.

Premanipulative testing with the lumbar spine held in full rotation stretch prior to the administration of the manipulative thrust will indicate if we have chosen the correct direction in which the manipulation should be performed. *In derangement this will always be in the direction that causes a decrease, centralisation or abolition of unilateral pain.* Reduction of symptoms may be achieved with the lumbar spine rotated either towards or away from the painful side. The deciding factor for the direction of the manipulation must be the reduction of mechanical deformation, irrespective of the fact whether this is achieved with movement towards or away from the painful side. *In dysfunction the patient should experience an enhancement of pain,* but the pain must never peripheralise. The patient with dysfunction may have to be manipulated in both directions, which is rarely the case in derangement.

A rotation manipulation is often described as having a gapping effect on the facet joints. Although this idea is widely held, it is almost impossible to detect on x-rays, taken during manipulation, that movement occurs at the facet joints. However, significant movement can be observed between the vertebral bodies. It is my contention that a rotation manipulation influences the nucleus and annulus of the disc more than the facet joints. Due to the torsion and side bending provided with the procedure, the annular wall must become tightened and under increased tension. This could possibly influence a distorted nucleus, at least as long as the annular wall is intact.

Manipulation consistently applied with the painful side uppermost in the belief that gapping of the facets is required to relieve the patient's symptoms, is no longer tenable. We must be guided by the increase and decrease of mechanical deformation instead of conjecture.

The term 'rotation manipulation' is perhaps incorrect, as there is a much greater side bending than rotation component when spinal rotation is performed.

Lightly built therapists who feel that they have inadequate weight to perform the rotation thrust procedure in flexion, can achieve equally satisfactory results by using the sustained rotation procedure.

PROCEDURE 13 — FLEXION IN LYING

The patient lies supine with the knees and hips flexed to about forty-five degrees and the feet flat on the couch. He bends the knees up towards the chest, firmly clasps the hands about them and applies overpressure to achieve maximum stress. The knees are then released and the feet placed back on the couch. The sequence is repeated about ten times. The first two or three flexion stresses are applied cautiously, but when the procedure is found to be safe the remaining pressures may become successively stronger, the last two or three being applied to the maximum possible (Fig. 8:13).

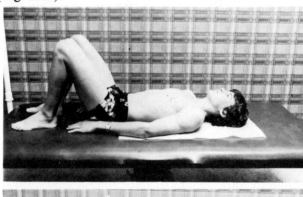

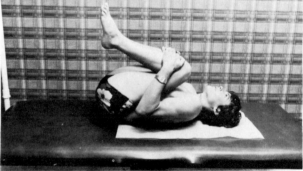

Fig. 8:13.
Flexion in lying.

Effects:

Flexion in lying causes a stretching of the posterior wall of the annulus, the posterior longitudinal ligament, the capsules of the facet joints, and other soft tissues. As the movement takes place from below upwards the lower lumbar and lumbo-sacral joints are placed on full stretch at the beginning of the exercise as soon as movement is initiated. Thus, the procedure is very important in flexion dysfunction when shortening of posterior soft tissues has occurred.

The procedure should *always be performed following stabilisation of a reduced posterior derangement*. This ensures that no flexion loss remains after the patient has become symptom free. By keeping the patient in extension and avoiding flexion as healing takes place, we permit scar formation with the joints in a shortened position. This shortened position will be held by the scar as it contracts, the patient remaining painfree but unable to flex. Any attempts to perform flexion beyond the limits imposed by the contracting scar, will produce pain. Therefore, further flexion will be avoided and adaptive shortening gradually worsens.

Flexion in lying performed regularly following reduction of posterior derangement allows the formation of an extensible scar in the midst of an elastic structure. Should we permit an inextensible scar to remain in the midst of an elastic structure, — the disc in this case — then sooner or later the patient will inadvertently move beyond the limitations of the scar, which results in further tearing of soft tissues and *apparent recurrence* of the derangement condition. This basic complication of healing exists throughout the muscular as well as the articular systems.

Flexion in lying also causes a posterior movement of the fluid nucleus and will be utilised in *anterior derangement situations* (Derangement seven) *to reverse the excessive anterior position of the nucleus.*

PROCEDURE 14 — FLEXION IN STANDING

The simple toe touching exercise in standing does not need much elaboration. The patient, standing with the feet about thirty centimeters apart, bends forward sliding the hands down the front of the legs in order to have some support and to measure the degree of flexion achieved. On reaching the maximum flexion allowed by pain or range, the patient returns to the upright position. The sequence is repeated about ten times, should be performed rhythmically, and initially with caution and without vigour. It is important to ensure that in between each movement the patient returns to neutral standing (Fig. 8:14).

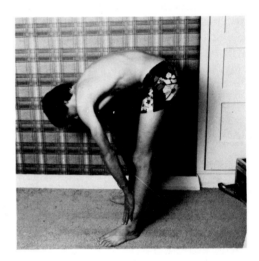

Fig. 8:14.
Flexion in standing.

Effects:

Flexion in standing differs from flexion in lying in various ways. Naturally, the gravitational and compressive forces act differently in both situations. In flexion in standing the movement takes place from above downwards, and the lower lumbar and lumbo-sacral joints are placed on full stretch only at the end of the movement. In addition, the lumbo-sacral nerve roots are pulled through the intervertebral foramina.

Thus, flexion in standing can be used as a progression of flexion in lying and may affect dysfunction as well as derangement. It can also be used specifically to stretch the scarring in an adherent nerve root or in nerve root entrapment.

If, in attempts to recover function following derangement, flexion in standing is performed too soon, the patient may rapidly worsen. This will happen even when there is no nerve root involvement. The same patient may safely perform flexion in lying and experience no increase in pain. It would appear that the gravitational stresses during flexion in standing are sufficient to cause an increase in derangement by further bulging of the disc wall.

Flexion in standing is an important procedure in the treatment of anterior derangement situations (Derangement Seven), as it causes a posterior movement of the nucleus within the disc wall.

PROCEDURE 15 — FLEXION IN STEP STANDING

In this procedure the patient stands on one leg while the other leg rests with the foot on a stool so that hip and knee are about ninety degrees flexed. Keeping the weight bearing leg straight the patient draws himself into a flexed position, firmly approximating the shoulder and the already raised knee (both being on the same side). If possible the shoulder should be moved even lower than the knee. The patient may apply further pressure by pulling on the ankle of the raised foot. The pressure is then released and the patient returns to the upright position. The sequence is repeated about six to ten times. It is important that the patient returns to neutral standing and restores the lordosis in between each movement (Fig. 8:15).

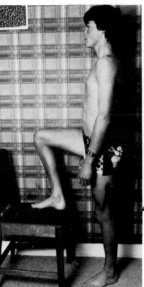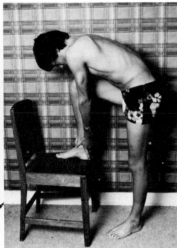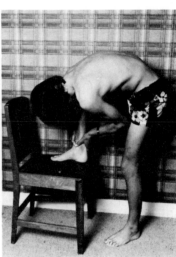

Fig. 8:15. *Flexion in step standing.*

Effects:

This procedure causes an asymmetrical flexion stress on the affected segments. It is applied when there is a deviation in flexion, which may occur in dysfunction as well as derangement. Both in dysfunction and derangement the leg to be raised is that opposite to the side to which the deviation in flexion is taking place — for example, in deviation in flexion to the left the right leg has to be raised.

In dysfunction asymmetrically shortened structures are stretched by flexion in step standing, provided it is performed often enough with the application of sufficient stress.

In derangement the procedure will influence the off-center nucleus so that it moves to a more central position, thus allowing the normal pathway of flexion to be regained. Where deviation in flexion is due to derangement some patients will experience a reversal of the deviation if the procedure is performed too often. Thus the exercise must be repeated only five to six times before checking if flexion in standing has been reduced to normal.

PROCEDURE 16 — CORRECTION OF LATERAL SHIFT

This procedure has two parts: first the deformity in scoliosis is corrected; then, if present, the deformity in kyphosis is reduced and full extension is restored.

The patient, standing with the feet about thirty centimeters apart, is asked to clearly define the areas where pain is being felt *at present*. The therapist stands on the side to which the patient is deviating and places the patient's near elbow at a right angle by his side. The elbow will be used to increase the lateral pressure against the patient's rib cage.

The therapist's arms encircle the patient's trunk, clasping the hands about the rim of the pelvis. Now the therapist presses his shoulder against the patient's elbow, pushing the patient's rib cage, thoracic and upper lumbar spine away while at the same time drawing the patient's pelvis towards himself. In this manner the deformity in scoliosis is reduced and, if possible slightly overcorrected.

Initially, there will be significant resistance to the procedure, which may actually cause an increase in pain. It is quite safe to continue with correction as long as centralisation of pain takes place, and therefore the patient must be questioned continually about the behaviour of his pain. Relaxation of the patient during the procedure is very important and we should always try to get the patient to 'let it all go'. The first pressure in the series should be a gentle gradual squeeze which is held momentarily and then released. After this an accurate assessment of the patient's reactions must be made. Experience has taught me that too much pressure or too fast a correction in the initial stages may result in fainting and collapse of the patient. If well tolerated the pressure is applied a little further each time. As correction progresses over ten to fifteen rhythmically applied pressures, the patient usually describes that the pain moves from a unilateral to a central position, and by the time over correction is achieved there will be a significant reduction in intensity of the pain or the pain may have moved slightly to the opposite side. If after a few rhythmical pressures no progress is made in the correction, it may be necessary to apply a longer and more sustained pressure.

Sometimes reduction may be felt clearly by the therapist and the patient's trunk is felt to move slowly but surely from its previously held position. In lightly-built or tall and slender patients shift correction may occur quite easily, and only a few minutes of ten to fifteen pressures are required to reduce the derangement. On the other hand, some acute lateral shifts are extremely difficult to reduce and one may have to perform five or six series of corrective pressures.

Assuming that correction of the deformity in scoliosis has been achieved, we must now proceed with restoring the lumbar lordosis. This is preferably commenced in the standing position. The patient no longer exhibits a lumbar scoliosis but may still have a kyphosis. The therapist, holding the patient as for correction of the scoliosis, must maintain slight over correction while moving the low back of the patient into the beginning of extension. A few movements will indicate the ease with which the lordosis will be restored. If the extension range improves rapidly it is usually better to recover as much extension as possible in the standing position. If extension does not increase rapidly, then it is better to change to extension in lying. This procedure should produce a steady and continuing reduction of central pain, and it should automatically follow for all patients with a postero-lateral derangement once the scoliosis has been corrected and the symptoms have centralised (Fig. 8:16).

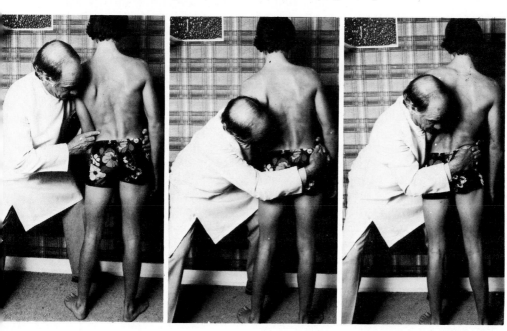

Fig. 8:16.
Correction of lateral shift.

Effects:

These will be discussed following the next procedure.

PROCEDURE 17 — SELF-CORRECTION OF LATERAL SHIFT

Having corrected the lateral shift and the blockage to extension, it is now *essential* to teach the patient to perform self-correction by side gliding in standing followed by extension in standing. This must be done on the very first day, so that the patient is equipped with a means of reducing the derangement himself at first sign of regression. Failure to teach self-correction will lead to recurrence within hours, ruining the initial reduction, and the patient will return the next day with the same deformity as on his first visit.

I have discarded the technique of self-correction as described previously[12] and instead I now teach patients to respond to pressures applied laterally against shoulder and pelvis. Initially, therapist' assistance is required. Patient and therapist stand facing each other. The therapist places one hand on the patient's shoulder on the side to which he deviates, and the other hand on the patient's opposite iliac crest. The therapist applies pressure by squeezing the patient between his hands, ensuring that the patient's shoulders remain parallel to the ground. When over correction has been achieved by the therapist, the mobility must be maintained by the patient who is therefore taught to actively respond to the pressures applied by the therapist. After some practise, remembering to keep the shoulders parallel to the ground, the heels on the ground and the knees straight, the patient can correct his own deformity. It is important to make the patient stand for a minute or two in the extreme over corrected position. Immediately following correction of the lateral deformity full extension must be restored. In the corrected standing position the patient must perform about ten repetitions of extension in standing.

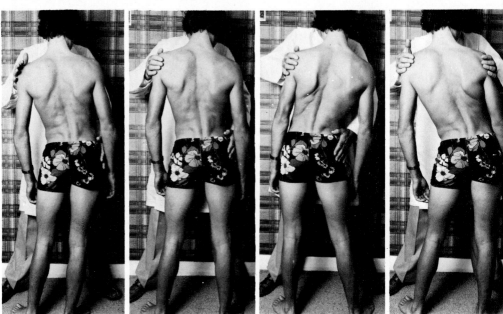

Fig. 8:17. *Self-correction of lateral shift.*

It must be emphasised that as long as the lordosis is retained there is little chance of recurrence of the derangement. If the patient is unable to maintain the reduction, he must perform self-correction during the day at regular intervals. The patient is advised to perform a series of extension in lying exercises after each session of self-correction (Fig. 8:17).

Effects and points to note:

It must be obvious that the last two procedures mainly influence the disc in derangement situations. In all instances time must be allowed for the reduction of the derangement to take place. Failure to correct the common lateral shift is usually the fault of the therapist, who has not taken enough time to allow a change in the contents of the disc to occur. The lateral shift correction including the restoration of extension must be an unhurried process and may take up to forty-five minutes in difficult patients. Constant repetition of the corrective procedures is necessary.

During the correction period there must be a continual reference to the patient's symptoms. When there is any suggestion of the production or enhancement of limb pain, treatment must be applied with great caution and a change should be made to the angle of flexion or extension in which the lateral shift is being corrected.

Maintenance of the lordosis following the reduction of the derangement must be emphasised from the first day, and we must ensure that the patient has adequate knowledge to retain his lordosis while sitting. The most common cause of regression or recurrence of symptoms within a few hours of reduction is a poor sitting posture. For example, after a successful reduction a patient may drive home for twenty to thirty minutes and on leaving the car full derangement has recurred. This occurs commonly and must be anticipated. In order to cope with this problem the patient should be provided with a lumbar support — for example, a rolled towel or something similar — to accentuate and support the lordosis in sitting.

In acute cases patients *should go home* (and not back to work) after reduction has been achieved. On arrival home they should move directly to a mirror and check if derangement has recurred. If so, they should perform the self-correction procedures before it becomes too difficult to reduce the lateral shift without outside help. Then they must lie prone for a few minutes on a bed or on the floor prior to performing a series of extension in lying exercises. This pattern should be repeated each hour or whenever possible throughout the day, and between exercise sessions the patient must be *lying and not sitting*. On retiring for bed the patient must lie supine in the over corrected position, with a lumbar support in the small of the back to maintain the lordosis, for about thirty minutes before going to sleep. The next morning there is usually a significant reduction in the deformity and pain after the correction procedure has been performed once or twice, although when first awaking the pain may be quite noticeable on movement.

Most patients with an acute lateral shift should be pain free in about seventy-two hours. A few difficult patients may take longer and many will take less time to reduce. Failure usually occurs because self-correction has not been taught adequately on the first visit.

Sciatic scoliosis with the complication of nerve root compression is more difficult to reduce than the uncomplicated lumbar scoliosis because the damage to the annulus is of such magnitude that outer fibres are distended. Reversal at this stage in the development of the derangement is always difficult. Treatment may also be rather difficult when patients have a lateral shift towards the painful side instead of the more common shift away from the pain. This may be because an escape of nuclear material has allowed the vertebral margins to approximate. Whatever the reason for this phenomenon, patients in this group are slow to progress and a few may completely fail to respond to treatment. Recovery can be so slow that one is never certain whether it is due to the treatment or just to the passage of time. Treatment procedures are the same as for patients who have a lateral shift away from the painful side, and the deformity must be corrected with due regard of the centralisation phenomenon. As in all cases, once the pain has resolved we must ensure that the function is restored, the posture is corrected and prophylaxis is taught.

There is a significantly higher incidence of sciatica in patients with a lateral shift towards the painful side and the incidence of failure to reductive measures is also higher in this group.

CHAPTER 9

The Postural Syndrome

DEFINITION

I would define the postural syndrome as mechanical deformation of postural origin causing pain of a strictly intermittent nature, which appears when the soft tissues surrounding the lumbar segments are placed under prolonged stress. This occurs when a person performs activities which keep the lumbar spine in a relatively static position (as in vacuuming, gardening) or when they maintain end positions for any length of time (as in prolonged sitting).

History

Patients with postural pain are usually aged thirty or under. Frequently they have a sedentary occupation and in general they lack physical fitness. In addition to low back pain they often describe pains in the mid-thoracic and cervical areas. They state that the pain is produced by positions and not by movement, is intermittent and may sometimes disappear for two to three days at a time. It is often found that, when patients are more active at weekends — playing tennis and dancing — they have relatively little or no trouble. The reason is that, although activity places more stress on the lumbar spine than does the adoption of static postures, with movement the stresses are continually changing and pain does not occur. The stresses arising from static postures, although less than those occuring during activity, are sustained and will, if maintained, eventually cause pain.

Examination

On examination no deformity is evident, no loss of movement will be detected and the test movements prove to be painfree. X-rays are normal and laboratory tests are negative. The patient's sitting and often the standing posture will be poor, and usually this is the only objective finding.

Clinical example

Let us look at the clinical example of a typical patient with the postural syndrome (Fig. 9:1). The patient has a bad posture indeed, and the pain cannot be reproduced by the test movements. To reproduce the appropriate postural stress, the patient must *assume and maintain* the position that is stated to cause pain — that is, the sitting posture. Only after the passage of sufficient time will

LUMBAR SPINE ASSESSMENT

Date.................. 29 FEBRUARY 1981
Name................. MARY SMITH
Address............. 24 OLD MILL ROAD
.... WELLINGTON
Date of birth.. 31 APRIL 1961
Occupation ..... SECRETARY

HISTORY

Symptoms now .... PAIN AT LUMBAR 3 4 5 CENTRALLY
.... ACROSS C7.T1 LATERALLY AND CENTRALLY T.56

at onset................
Present for..... 8 MONTHS
Commenced as a result of,...
No apparent reason. ☑
~~Constant~~/Intermittent.

When worse —   bending,   sitting ~~or rising from,~~ ✓   standing, ✓   walking,   lying.
Other.............. AT END OF DAY
When better —   bending,   sitting or rising from,   standing,   walking, ✓   lying. ✓
Other .... IN A.M. AND WHEN ACTIVE ESPECIALLY AT WEEKENDS

Disturbed sleep — ~~Yes~~   No   Cough/sneeze ~~+ve~~ —ve
.... NIL
Previous history..............
   and treatment..............
X-Rays .... OK
General health .... OK   Meds/Steroids .... NIL
Recent surgery .... NIL   Accident............ NO
Gait .... OK   Bladder .... OK

EXAMINATION

Posture sitting .... POOR
Posture standing........ POOR   Lordosis ~~reduced~~/accentuated............
Lateral shift ~~(R) or (L)~~ or nil   Leg length .... OK

MOVEMENT LOSS   NIL

Flexion: Major.   Moderate.   Minimal.   Deviation (R) or (L)............ OK
Extension: Major.   Moderate.   Minimal.   Deviation (R) or (L)............ OK
Side Gliding: (R) or (L) ....

TEST MOVEMENTS

FIS.. NO PAIN PRODUCED   SGIS (R)...... NO PAIN
REP. FIS "   "   "   SGIS (L) .... "   "
EIS .. "   "   "   REP. SGIS (R)........ "   "
REP. EIS .. "   "   "   REP. SGIS (L) ....
FIL .. "   "   "   UNABLE TO PRODUCE PAIN WITH MOVEMENT.
REP. FIL .. "   "   "   PAIN PRODUCED AFTER ½ HOUR SITTING SLOUCHED.
EIL .. "   "   "   PAIN ABOLISHED ON POSTURAL CORRECTION.
REP. EIL..............
Neurological .... OK
Hip joints................ OK   S.I.   OK
Conclusion: Posture   ~~Dysfunction~~   ~~Derangement~~

PRINCIPLE OF TREATMENT   POSTURE CORRECTION SITTING AND STANDING
PROPHYLAXIS

the symptoms appear in this position, and up to half an hour may be required before pain is felt. Once pain has been produced by adoption of a certain posture, it will be abolished by correction of that posture. Now our suspicions are confirmed and a diagnosis can be made. In short, the patient with the postural syndrome has no clinical or laboratory findings indicating a particular pathology and all functions appear perfectly normal.

Thousands of people are seeking treatment for pain resulting from bad postures; they consult doctors who often are unsuited to deal with the problem and, taking the easiest way out, prescribe pain relieving drugs instead of recommending postural correction; disillusioned with drug therapy patients attend a chiropractor, osteopath, physiotherapist or some fringe manipulator who, mainly out of ignorance, proceeds to manipulate joints in which there is no pathology and certainly nothing 'out of place'.

I must emphasise that in many patients presenting with postural pain no pathology needs to exist. All patients with low back pain have an increase in pain when postural stresses are added. In derangement and dysfunction there is a pathological cause for the pain, and postural stresses may enhance the pathological state. *But in the postural syndrome no pathology is present,* and the *only treatment that is required is postural correction and re-education and instruction in prophylaxis.*

Postures involved

Every patient with pain of postural origin has a different description for the circumstances leading to the production of pain. Sitting (Fig. 9:2), by no means

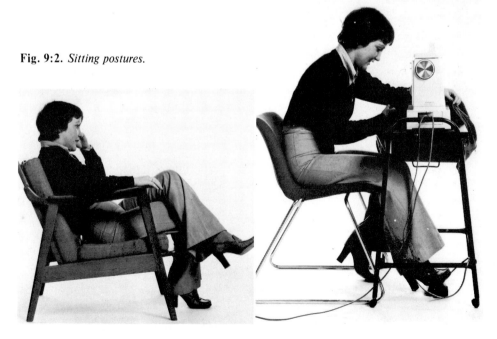

Fig. 9:2. *Sitting postures.*

Fig. 9:1. (opposite) *Clinical example of a typical patient with the postural syndrome.*

the only postural situation causing and prolonging low back pain, is the most frequent cause of postural pain. Some patients will name the sitting position purely and simply as causative, and they complain that pain is produced as soon as they spend more than a certain amount of time, say ten minutes, in any sort of chair or car seat. Others will describe sitting at the typewriter as the only time that pain is felt. Bus, taxi, and car drivers all complain of being worse while seated for long periods in their vehicles; both pilots and passengers complain about the seating in airplanes.

Working in prolonged standing positions also may cause postural pain, but the opportunity to move and change position is greater in standing than in sitting and the avenues for relief are more numerous. Consequently, there are less complaints of pain arising from the standing position than from sitting. People who work in cramped positions, be it standing or sitting, are also likely to complain of low back pain. The incidence of low back pain is very high in people who work in continuously stooped positions (Fig. 9:3).

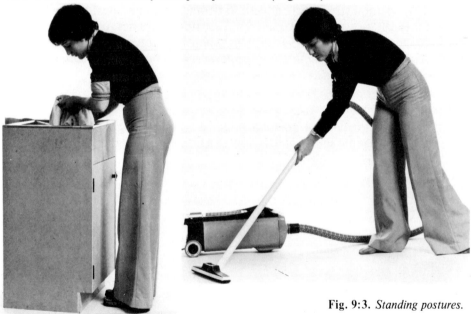

Fig. 9:3. *Standing postures.*

The lying position (Fig. 9:4) may be an additional source of stress enhancing low back pain, and if pain predominantly occurs while lying it requires thorough investigation.

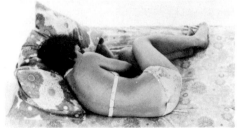

Fig. 9:4.
Lying posture.

TREATMENT OF THE POSTURAL SYNDROME

Every patient must be examined and analysed individually, and educated for his own particular postural stress. Education is probably the most important part of the treatment for low back pain of postural origin. The patient must have a clear and unambiguous explanation of the mechanism that produces his pain. He must realise that, when he assumes the positions of stress causing pain, he is in fact pulling the ligaments apart; and all that is required to stop his postural pain, is to stop stressing the ligaments for about ten days. I also explain to the patient that once he commences the correction regime, he *will and should* develop some new pains which are commonly felt higher in the back. This is merely the consequence of adjustment to a new postural habit.

The more often pain is triggered, the more readily it will occur. And the less often pain is triggered, the more difficult it is to be produced. Thus, poor sitting positions maintained regularly will cause pain after the passage of less and less time. Conversely, good sitting postures will enable the patient to remain pain free for longer and longer periods, and when slouching next occurs it will take much more time for the pain to arise. After two weeks of correct sitting patients will be able to slouch for short periods without having pain. However, no one should be permitted to slouch for extended periods. For example, a patient who usually gets low back pain after ten minutes of slouched sitting, may after a couple of weeks of sitting correctly revert to the slouched position and only experience pain after twenty minutes in that position. This painfree slouched sitting period can be progressed up to a limit, so that at the end of ten weeks of correct sitting a patient may well be able to slouch for an hour or two. A possible explanation for this phenomenon is forthcoming from Professor P. D. Wall.[35]

Correction of the sitting posture

All patients who have low back pain produced or enhanced by prolonged sitting, should receive an adequate explanation regarding the cause of pain and the need for maintenance of the correct sitting posture.

We must explain that when a person sits his spine will sooner or later take up a relaxed posture. Unless a special lumbar support is given or a conscious effort is made to maintain the lordosis, the lumbar spine will move into a fully flexed position placing various ligamentous structures on full stretch. The nucleus of the intervertebral discs is forced posteriorly, the intradiscal pressure rises, and the stresses on the posterior wall of the annulus are increased. At this stage there are many reasons for the spine to feel *uncomfortable*. If this position is maintained for a long period, the spine will become *painful* as well and in some cases derangement may occur. Few patients fail to comprehend our explanations, provided these are couched in terms understandable to the layman.

To convince the patient that our suspicions about his sitting posture are correct it is necessary to prove this to him. Pain of postural origin arising by sitting incorrectly will be abolished by sitting correctly. During the first treatment session we must reproduce the pain by positioning the patient and allowing enough time for postural stresses to build up. Once pain is felt the patient is easily convinced that it is posture-related, when on adopting the correct sitting posture the pain ceases. If we cannot reproduce the symptoms during the first treatment, we must instruct the patient to assess the relationship between posture and pain himself by correction of the sitting posture the next time pain is felt.

To achieve correction of the sitting posture the following is necessary:

(1) firstly the patient must *be able to obtain* the correct sitting posture;

(2) then he must *know how to maintain* it when sitting for prolonged periods.

To obtain the correct sitting posture

The patient must have a good understanding of the correct sitting posture, and his control of the muscles and joints involved in obtaining it must be restored. Therefore, it is necessary that he be acquainted with the extreme of the good and bad sitting positions before he is instructed regarding the correct sitting posture.

In order to achieve this we have to introduce *the 'slouch-overcorrect' procedure*. The patient must sit slouched on a backless chair or stool, allow the lumbar spine to rest on the ligaments in the fully flexed position, and permit head and chin to protrude. Then he must smoothly move into the erect sitting posture with the *lordosis at its maximum* and the head held directly over the spine with the chin pulled in. This sequence should be repeated in a flowing rhythmical manner, so that the patient moves *from the extreme of the good to the extreme of the bad position* (Fig. 9:5).

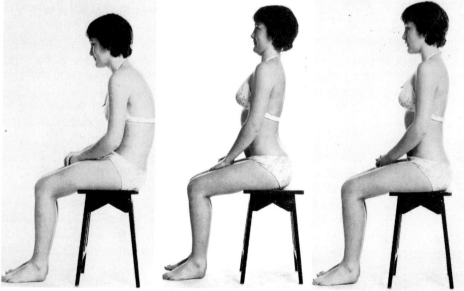

Fig. 9:5a.
Slouched sitting.

Fig. 9:5b.
Overcorrected sitting.

Fig. 9:5c.
Correct sitting.

Figures 5a and b together form the 'slouch-overcorrect' procedure, and Figure 5c shows the ten percent release from the overcorrected position.

After some practise at this most patients are able to find the extreme of the good sitting position. They should become so good at it, that at the snap of the fingers they can assume the overcorrected sitting posture and hold it for a few minutes. Once this can be achieved patients are advised to follow this procedure whenever pain is felt and to maintain the extreme of the good sitting position for a few minutes. Pain induced by poor sitting is nearly always quickly abolished by this method. On discovering the relationship between sitting postures and pain by this simple exercise few patients fail to carry out our advice. Postural correction and exercises related to pain are easily understood and performed by most people.

Once the patient has a good understanding of the good and bad postures he can assume while sitting, he must be taught which position is *the correct sitting posture*. The extreme of the good position is of course closest to the desirable, but it is impossible to hold this position for any length of time because various structures are on full stretch and will become painful with time. Therefore, the patient is instructed to move into the extreme of lordosis and then release the last ten percent of the movement. After this release from fully strained erect sitting the position can easily be maintained if necessary. This is the position that must be adopted habitually in the future. It must be emphasised that in the correct sitting posture the lumbar spine always has a certain amount but not the maximum of lordosis. If postural pain arises in the sitting position, it is caused by an insufficient or lost lordosis and postural correction will abolish the pain.

Thus, in order to learn how to assume the correct sitting posture with a lumbar lordosis patients must be instructed to carry out the 'slouch-overcorrect' procedure three times daily, fifteen to twenty times at each session. At the end of each session they must release the last ten percent of the extreme good sitting position. They have now found the correct sitting posture. This routine must be kept up for three to four days at least, longer if necessary, until the correct posture becomes automatic.

To maintain the correct sitting posture

When sitting for prolonged periods it is *essential that a certain amount of lordosis be maintained at all times*. From the very first day the patient must be shown how this can be achieved. The lumbar spine may be held in lordosis in two ways:

(a) actively by conscious control of the lordosis, when sitting on a seat without backrest.

(b) passively by the use of a lumbar support, when sitting on a seat with a backrest. The purpose of the lumbar supportive roll is to hold the lumbar spine in a good but not extreme lordosis in the sitting position while relaxing, working and driving the car. Without the support the lordosis will be lost as soon as a person leans back in a chair or concentrates on anything other than maintaining the lordosis.

The lumbar roll as sitting support:

A roll inserted in the small of the back provides adequate support for the lumbar spine in sitting, provided the apex of the support maintains the lordosis just short of its maximum. When placed at or just above the belt line, affecting approximately the area of the third and fourth lumbar vertebrae, it produces the optimum lordosis, provided one sits with the sacrum against the back of the chair (Fig. 9:6). A cushion is not a suitable lumbar support because, when placed behind the low back, it merely pushes the whole spine a few centimeters away from the back of the chair without in any way influencing the angle of extension or degree of lordosis in the lumbar spine.

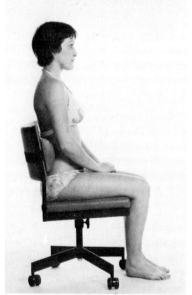

Fig. 9:6a.
Use of lumbar roll in office chair.

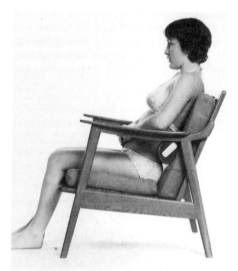

Fig. 9:6b.
Use of lumbar roll in easy chair. This roll can also be used for support in a car seat.

Various rolls can be made for the different situations in which they may be required — for example, lounge chair, office chair and car seat. If a lounge chair or car seat is designed in such a way that the roll is absorbed by the upholstery, it may be necessary to place one or more cushions in the chair first and then add the lumbar roll.

Patients frequently complain about the effort they must expend to maintain the correct sitting posture, more so when this is done actively than with the help of a lumbar roll. In fact, many patients will describe a strain pain or say that the new position is a painful one. It is important that these pains are recognised as new postural stresses *which should normally occur*. If after a day or two of correct sitting a patient has not complained of 'new pains', it is likely that he has not maintained the corrected position often and long enough. Adjustment to a new posture results in shortlived transitional aching of a different quality and location than the pain which initially forced consultation. It should not last longer than five to six days.

It is reported[22] that most people in North America sit with the lumbar lordosis accentuated. On several visits to the United States and Canada I have had the pleasure of treating some hundreds of patients, and I was relieved to notice that most of these, as well as most of the doctors and physiotherapists attending my courses, sat with the lumber spine held in flexion after about half an hour of sitting. I was relieved because I had been wondering whether patients in North America just might be different from those in Australasia and Europe, in which case the treatments I have developed would be most unsuitable in the North American continent. I mention this to draw attention to a fundamental error in the clinical observation of the basic mechanics of the sitting posture, which has led to the development of an inflexible concept of treatment for low back pain throughout North America based on the assumption that the lordosis is undesirable, extension harmful and flexion beneficial.

In that continent, the treatment of low back pain has been influenced by authors who argue that damage in the posterior compartment of the disc is the result of compressive forces exerted by the lordotic posture which they believe is a predominant feature of western cultures. The treatment recommended involves a combination of flexion exercises and postures all carefully calculated to reduce the lumbar lordosis. Supporters of the flexion philosophy argue that African and Asian cultures do not have as high an incidence of back pain as is found in western society and this is largely because of the flexed spinal postures adopted by these cultures. Other authorities, Armstrong,[14] and more recently Hickey and Hukins,[43] state that annular failure under compression is unlikely to be a significant cause of low back pain. White and Panjabi[44] were not aware of any investigation in which cross cultural and racial comparisons had ever been satisfactorily studied and related to low back pain. They also state that Williams flexion exercises are based on the assumption that achieving and maintaining a flexed lumbar spine is preferable, but "this has not been proved and is contrary to evidence of studies in vivo of intradiscal pressure and electromyographic studies".[44]

Another widespread misconception, held by many doctors and therapists, suggests that postural correction can be achieved by strengthening the muscles of the spine. Strengthening of muscles has no effect on posture. No strengthening exercises will educate muscles to maintain the correct posture. Actively maintaining the correct posture is the only way to achieve postural correction. This has the added bonus that the muscles required to maintain this position are automatically strengthened merely by performing the task for which they were originally designed.

In postural retraining the problem does not lie in the inability to assume the correct posture, but in a loss of awareness of the correct posture, if indeed such an awareness existed. To restore this it is necessary to retrain postural concepts, which is essentially a matter of the will. Indeed, willpower motivated by pain must be our tool. We are able to show the patient what must be done to correct his posture, but only he himself can do it.

Correction of the standing posture

Prolonged standing is another position in which low back pain may be enhanced. Usually, the patient can be seen to stand with a protruding abdomen and the lordosis at its extreme, 'hanging' on the lumbo-sacral ligaments. To achieve postural correction in standing the patient must be shown how to move the lower part of the spine backwards by tightening the abdominal muscles and tilting the pelvis backwards, while at the same time moving the upper spine forwards and raising the chest (Fig. 9:7).

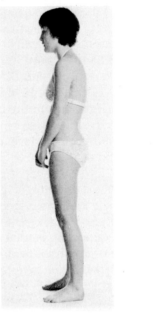
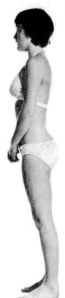

Fig. 9:7a. (right)
Relaxed standing.

Fig. 9:7b. (far right)
Correct standing.

There are two common relaxed standing positions. One is achieved simply by folding one's arms and allowing the chest to drop. Chest and thoracic spine move posteriorly and pelvis moves anteriorly. This places the lower lumbar and lumbo-sacral joints into full extension. You can try this for yourself and will find that, once having adopted this position further movement into extension is impossible. The best way to observe if this posture is the cause of the patient's pain, is to talk with him for some time until he is standing relaxed. If pain is present due to this position, correction should reduce or abolish it.

To re-educate a patient with this stance, we must first place him in the relaxed standing position until pain is produced. Alteration of the angle of pelvic inclination will reduce the standing pain almost immediately. This is best achieved by lifting the chest and thoracic spine, simultaneously tilting the pelvis slightly backwards. The ability to control the pelvic inclination in standing must be mastered first; then the angle at which the pain is abolished must be established and maintained. If pain in standing can not be reproduced on the first examination the patient must be instructed to evaluate the relationship between posture and pain himself by postural correction the next time pain is felt.

The second relaxed standing position is obtained by taking all the body weight on one leg, while the knee of the other leg is allowed to bend causing the pelvis to droop at the same side. The lumbar spine moves into a full side gliding/rotation position. Again, you can try this for yourself and will find that having adopted this position no further movement into side gliding or extension is possible. If this position produces pain it is easily corrected and avoidance of the standing habit should suffice.

Correction of the lying posture

Pain in the lying position is common. It causes considerable distress when it interferes with sleep over a long enough period, and it requires attention when the patient regularly wakes up with pain in the morning, the pain abating as the day progresses. There are two factors to be investigated:

(a) The lying posture itself. This is different for each person and must be dealt with individually. The lying posture during sleep is difficult to influence.

(b) The surface on which one is lying. For the majority of people the mattress itself should not be too hard, whereas the base on which the mattress rests must be firm and unyielding. This allows adequate support for the contours of the body without placing stresses on the spine. Usually, the surface on which one is lying is easily corrected or modified.

When dealing with pain produced by lying in bed, I have three recommendations to make which may be worth considering:

Due to the natural contours of the body — that is, wider at shoulders and pelvis than at the waist — and due to the lordotic curvature of the lumbar spine, the lumbar area may be placed under stress in the prone, supine or side lying position. This is particularly so when a hard mattress is supported by a firm and unyielding base. If this is thought to be the cause of the problem, the patient should use a lumbar supportive roll. When lying prone the roll will prevent extreme extension in the lumbar spine. When lying supine with the legs outstretched the roll will fill the gap between the lumbar spine and the mattress and prevent sagging of the spine into flexion. When lying on the side it will fill the gap between pelvis and ribs and prevent sagging of the spine into side bending. This type of lumbar support in bed usually works quickly or not at all, and should be tried for about three nights.

The lumbar roll as lying support

A beach towel folded end to end and then rolled cross-wise usually fits around the average middle. If this is too big a bath towel folded length-wise can be used instead. Each patient will have to experiment to find the correct size of lumbar roll required in his particular case. He should wrap the towel around the belt line and attach the two ends to each other. If left loose the roll will not remain in place and may, when positioned anywhere else than at the waist, further increase the stresses placed on the spine (Fig. 9:8).

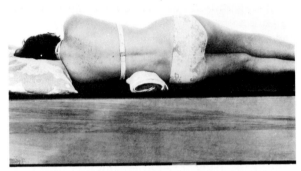

Fig. 9:8.
Use of lumbar roll in lying. The roll is not fastened in the picture in order to show the shape of the spine.

When the base of the mattress is not firm enough or the mattress itself is too soft, stresses may also be placed on the lumbar spine. Because of the costs involved in replacing a mattress or its base, I always recommend that the mattress be placed on the floor if it is felt that a firm flat base is required. If there is no improvement after sleeping three to four nights on a flat surface, it is unlikely that this is the answer to the patient's problems.

There is a small number of people who require a sagging mattress. Usually these people fall under the flexion principle category. The sagging mattress can easily be created by placing pillows at both ends of the bed in between the mattress and its base to form a dish shape.

Conclusion

We should now have equipped the patient with sufficient information enabling him to sensibly control mechanical stresses and deal with symptoms himself. The essence of treatment of the postural syndrome is that, *if it is possible for patients to stop their pain, it is also possible for them to prevent the onset of the pain.* I feel that it is negligent of the medical and physiotherapy professions to continue giving relief for episodic pain without familiarising patients with the manner in which their pain arises and providing them with the means to prevent the onset of such pain. It is my experience that patients with postural pain, when properly instructed and advised, treat themselves ably and adequately. They can well control their postural stresses, and only need assistance when excessive and sometimes unexpected external forces have been placed on their joints — for example, following lifting heavy weights, stepping unexpectedly from the pavement, being hit by a motor vehicle, a sudden bout of coughing or sneezing while sitting or bent forwards.

When treatment is completed successfully we must explain to the patient that, although the present pain has been relieved, recurrence of similar symptoms is possible whenever he forgets postural care for extended periods. The consequences of postural neglect should be discussed when appropriate.

Consequences of postural neglect

The effects of postural habits on the shape of man are obvious when we observe people around us. If head and chin are allowed to protrude long and often enough, the ability to glide the head dorsally will be lost which results in a permanently protruding head and a dowager's hump. As age advances this once reversible situation will become irreversible. People with this type of posture have a flattened lumbar spine as well, and by the age of seventy the ability to stand erect is lost so that they walk with a slight stoop. Movement that was once easily obtained is lost forever. But this postural stoop is not the inevitable consequence of ageing. Loss of function can be prevented if movements in the desired direction are performed adequately and often enough.

Initially, poor postural habits will only produce pain without loss of function. If as a result of continuous slouched sitting, flexion is regularly performed but extension never, the anterior structures of the joints involved will shorten and the posterior structures will lengthen. In this way flexion remains readily obtainable, but extension becomes more and more difficult and will therefore be avoided. Thus, the consequences of postural neglect are adaptive shortening leading to dysfunction.

Adaptive shortening implies loss of function and movement. In addition to the production of pain whenever the shortened structures are placed on stress, this loss of movement and function must inevitably lead to impairment of nutrition in an avascular structure like the disc. This will become one of the contributing factors of disc degeneration.

We should point out to people engaged in sedentary occupations that adaptive shortening and dysfunction due to poor posture can be prevented by regular postural correction and adequate performance of the appropriate exercises before adaptive shortening is allowed to develop.

TYPICAL TREATMENT PROGRESSION —
THE POSTURAL SYNDROME

The days referred to in the treatment progression are related to treatment sessions which do not necessarily take place on consecutive days. This also applies for the treatment progressions of the dysfunction and derangement syndromes.

Day one

— Assessment and conclusion/diagnosis.
— Postural discussion ensuring adequate explanation of the nature of the problem. The patient must understand the cause of pain. I usually give the simple example of pain arising from the passively bent forefinger.
— We must satisfy ourselves and the patient that the pain can be induced and abolished by positioning. If it is not possible to induce pain during the first treatment session, the patient must be instructed mow to abolish pain by postural correction when next it appears.

— Commence with postural correction exercises and give postural advice; do not try to teach too much the first visit.
— Discuss the importance of maintenance of the lordosis while sitting prolonged, and demonstrate the use of lumbar supports in sitting and lying.

Day two

— Confirm diagnosis.
— Check results. If the patient was unsuccessful in controlling the postural pain on his own, it is possible that we have not taught correction well enough. It also may be that the patient has not corrected his posture adequately or maintained the corrected posture long enough. When confronted with such a suggestion in an accusing manner, patients often feel offended and deny having slouched. We must be tactful when discussing these points.
— If possible have the patient produce and abolish the pain; otherwise enquire as to his ability to abolish the pain during the preceeding twenty-four hours by correcting the posture whenever pain appeared.
— Check the exercises. It is surprising how often patients alter the exercises without realising it.
— Repeat the postural advice in full.
— Inform the patient that 'new pains' are to be expected as a result of adjustment to different postural habits.

Day three

— Treatment as for day two.
— Once the patient is adequately controlling his postural stresses, treatment may be altered from a daily basis to every second or third day.
— Once the pain occurs only occasionally and can be well controlled, the patient may stop the 'slouch-overcorrect' exercise.
— Reassure regarding the onset of 'new' postural pains.

Day four and five

— Check exercises and progress.
— Deal with any other postural pain that may have become apparent.
— Deal with other situations which may have previously been overlooked.

Further treatments

— A few check-ups at greater intervals may be necessary to ensure the patient has full control of his postural pain.
— We must ensure that the patient has adequately stressed the joints and is engaged in all normal activities.
— Discuss the consequences of postural neglect.
— Before discharge prophylaxis must be discussed in detail.

CHAPTER 10

The Dysfunction Syndrome

The word 'dysfunction' chosen by Mennell[36] to describe the loss of movement commonly known as 'joint play' or 'accessory movement' seems infinitely preferable to the terms 'osteopathic lesion' and 'chiropractic subluxation', neither of which means anything and both of which mean everything. 'Dysfunction' or 'not functioning correctly' at least acknowledges that something is wrong without going through the sham procedure of pretending that only those who belong to the club really understand the terminology. For years osteopaths and chiropractors have claimed that only the people, properly trained in their particular calling, have the necessary knowledge to understand their terminology. There may be some truth in that.

Although I believe that the term 'dysfunction' as used by Mennell[36] does not strictly cover the loss of movement caused by adaptive shortening, I have chosen to use this term instead of repeatedly referring to 'adaptive shortening'.

Essentially, the mechanism of pain production in dysfunction is the same as in normal tissues — that is, when overstretching of soft tissues causes sufficient mechanical deformation of the free nerve endings in these tissues, pain will arise. In dysfunction soft tissues in or around the segment involved are shortened or contain contracted scar tissue. When normal movement is attempted these structures are placed on full stretch somewhat prematurely. While normally movement in the joint would take place over a certain distance before being stopped by ligamentous tension, it is now brought to a halt after only part of that distance is completed. Attempts to move further towards end range will result in overstretching and produce pain. The pain is felt at the end of the existing range and ceases immediately after end range stretch is released. Repeated uncontrolled stretching of contracted soft tissues will lead to further micro-traumata and pain. The patient then avoids the movement which is painful, and adaptive shortening of the scar reduces the existing range of movement even more.

DEFINITION

Developed as a result of poor postural habit, spondylosis, trauma or derangement, the dysfunction syndrome is the condition in which adaptive shortening and resultant loss of mobility causes pain prematurely — that is, before achievement of full normal end range movement. Essentially, the condition arises because movement is performed inadequately at a time that contraction of soft tissues is taking place.

95

History

There are two possibilities regarding the cause of dysfunction. When dysfunction develops following trauma or derangement, the patient will be aware of the onset. He will describe the symptoms from the date of trauma or derangement, but the pain produced by trauma or derangement will no longer be present and the symptoms are now related to the resultant loss of mobility and function. When dysfunction is the result of poor posture or spondylosis the patient will be unaware of the onset. He will be unable to relate the cause of the pain to a particular incident and usually describes a gradual slow onset of pain commencing for no apparent reason.

Patients in the dysfunction category are likely to be over thirty years of age. However, younger patients may well present, who have had previous low back pain or trauma which resulted in loss of function that has not been detected or treated.

The pain is felt at the end range of certaincmovements, or before end range is achieved, and this may interfere with the performance of simple tasks. For example, loss of function in the neck is often first noticed when the motorist turns the head while reversing the car; in loss of function in the low back it is often difficult to put stockings on the feet or to get into the trousers.

Initially patients with dysfunction are stiff first thing in the morning, loosening as the day progresses. But as time passes flexion and extension become reduced and the morning stiffness does not pass. In extension dysfunction lying prone for any length of time — for example, on the beach — cannot be tolerated. Due to inadequate extension in the lumbar spine the ligamentous structures are placed on full stretch prematurely while lying prone and pain is produced.

Often the patient with dysfunction states that he feels better when he is active and moving about than when at rest. The reasons for this are obvious: during regular and not excessive activity end range of movement is seldom required and, if so, only momentarily; on the other hand, during resting end positions are readily assumed and as soon as they are maintained they may prove painful.

In dysfunction the pain is intermittent, occurring only when periarticular structures are placed on full stretch. This happens much sooner in a patient with dysfunction than in a normal person, hence the much more frequent provocation of pain in dysfunction. The greater the loss of function, the more often will the pain occur.

Pain from dysfunction sometimes develops in an episodic manner and appears to resemble derangement. This episodic pain is triggered by excessive use, for example a vigorous afternoon in the garden. Overstretching of contracted soft tissues causes minor traumata and produces or increases pain. If the patient rests for a few days the pain subsides, but further scarring and healing contractures will increasingly limit the available range of movement. This becomes a vicious circle which will only be broken by treatment procedures as described for dysfunction.

Examination

Generally, the posture of the patient with dysfunction will be poor. In the absence of trauma or previous back pain episodes, often only poor posture is to be blamed for the development of dysfunction. This is confirmed by merely correcting the posture which relieves the patient of a significant amount of pain.

Except in the elderly with dysfunction, deformity is not commonly seen. However, there is always a loss of movement or function. Often the loss of movement is a capsular pattern type of restriction. This is clearly described by Cyriax[24] for spinal as well as peripheral joints. When dysfunction in the spine is the result of poor posture or spondylosis, there tends to be a symmetrical movement loss in all directions and group lesions are commonly seen. However, when dysfunction is the result of trauma and derangement there is more often an asymmetrical movement loss, some movements remaining full range and others being partially or completely lost. Group lesions may or may not develop following trauma depending on the extent of the damage sustained, and are hardly ever seen following derangement.

If there is a significant loss of extension, (Fig. 10:1) the lordosis may be reduced or the patient may be unable to produce the lordosis, even if he strains to do so. If there is a loss of flexion, (Fig. 10:2) the patient may have difficulty in reaching his toes and on bending forwards the lumbar spine may remain in slight lordosis. Alternatively, the loss of flexion may become apparent midway through the flexion excursion by a deviation of the body to one side or other of the midline (Fig. 10:3). Many variables are possible and all must be noted in order to determine the pattern of movement restriction of each patient individually.

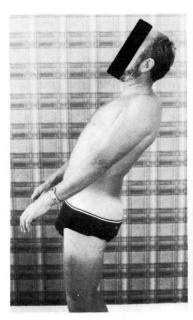
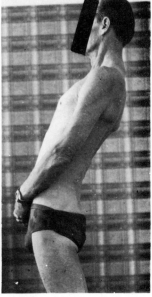

Fig. 10:1.
Loss of extension.

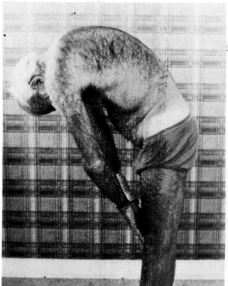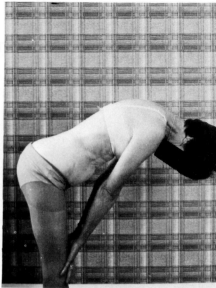

Fig. 10:2. *Loss of flexion.*

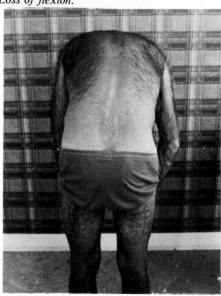

Fig. 10:3.
Loss of flexion with deviation.

The test movements

It will not be difficult to reproduce the symptoms with the test movements. Due to the reduced end range of some movements pain is elicited readily as soon as stretching of these movements is performed, and each time the stress is released the pain subsides quickly.

Following the test movements the patient should be allowed to move about and perhaps have a short walk. The object of this is to determine the effect of the test movements on the general pain pattern. A patient with dysfunction may be slightly more aware of his pain after the examination, but he will *never remain significantly worse, provided tissue damage due to overstretching of shortened structures has not taken place.* Following the test movements the movement pattern will not have altered — that is, if we were to repeat the whole sequence the same movements would produce the same pain as in the first session.

Clinical example

Let us look at the example of a typical patient with dysfunction (Fig. 10:4). In particular we must assess the effects of the test movements on the pain. In this patient pain is produced at the point of full stretch in flexion and extension, which are both restricted in range of movement. Repetition of the test movements does not make the symptoms better or worse, and on release of the stress the pain subsides leaving the patient no worse than before testing. *Rapid changes of symptoms do not occur in dysfunction.* It takes weeks for soft tissues to become contracted and adaptively shortened and, likewise, it will take a long time for them to lengthen again.

Treatment of the dysfunction syndrome

Patients who fall in the dysfunction category will still require postural instruction. When planning treatment we must include from the first day *all* the procedures laid down for the patient with postural pain. The patient with dysfunction can learn quickly to control those symptoms which are caused or enhanced by bad posture.

The symptoms of dysfunction are more related to movement and become evident in the difficulty or inability of the patient to accomplish end range of movement, most noticeable in the extremes of flexion and extension. These symptoms will remain present until the length of the shortened tissues is increased and the range of movement is improved. This will be achieved in about four to six weeks, provided the treatment procedures are used in a precise and clearly defined manner. The *very nature of adaptive shortening of soft tissues adjacent to articular structures prohibits the rapid recovery of function in a few days.*

Stretching must be performed in such a way that it allows elongation of ligamentous structures and scar tissue without causing micro-traumata. Pain produced by stretching should stop shortly after the stress is released. When pain persists long after stretching has occurred *overstretching* has taken place.

To achieve lengthening of soft tissues it is not sufficient to perform stretching once a week, neither is it sufficient to do this once a day. Too many physiotherapy clinics make their patients return daily for ten minutes of mobilisation or, worse still, one minute of manipulation with the express purpose of restoring mobility. This concept of treatment may well be acceptable, if the patient is given adequate exercises to perform regularly in between treatment sessions. However, often enough this is not done; or else, when the

LUMBAR SPINE ASSESSMENT

Date .... 29 FEBRUARY 1981
Name .... BILL SMITH
Address .... 24 OLD MILL ROAD
.... WELLINGTON
Date of birth . 31 APRIL 1939
Occupation .... CARPENTER

HISTORY

Symptoms now .... ACROSS L4.5

at onset .... SAME
Present for .... FOUR MONTHS
Commenced as a result of ....
No apparent reason. ☑
Constant/Intermittent.   ✔   ✔
When worse —   bending,   sitting ~~or rising from,~~   standing,   walking,   PRONE lying. ✔
Other .... FIRST THING A.M.
When better —   bending,   sitting or rising from,   standing, ✔   walking, ✔   SUPINE lying. ✔
Other .... WHEN MOVING
Disturbed sleep — ~~Yes~~   No   Cough/sneeze ~~+ve~~ —ve
Previous history ...... RECURRING EPISODIC LOW BACK PAIN 10 YRS. 8X
and treatment .... NIL
X-Rays .... MINOR DEGENERATIVE CHANGES AT L45 — 5.SI
General health .... GOOD   Meds/Steroids .... NO
Recent surgery .... NO   Accident .... NO
Gait .... OK   Bladder .... OK

EXAMINATION

Posture sitting .... NOT GOOD   Lordosis reduced/~~accentuated~~ ....
Posture standing ...... GOOD   Leg length .... OK
Lateral shift (~~R) or (L)~~ or nil

MOVEMENT LOSS

Flexion: ~~Major.~~   ~~Moderate.~~   Minimal.   Deviation (R) or (L) .... NO
Extension: Major.   ~~Moderate.~~   ~~Minimal.~~   Deviation (R) or (L) .... NO
Side Gliding: (R) or (L) ....   Reduced or O.K. .... OK

TEST MOVEMENTS

FIS PRODUCES PAIN AT END RANGE	SGIS (R)	OK
REP. FIS " " DOES NOT WORSEN	SGIS (L)	OK
EIS " " AT END RANGE	REP. SGIS (R)	OK
REP. EIS " " BUT DOES NOT WORSEN	REP. SGIS (L)	OK
FIL OK		
REP. FIL OK		
EIL PRODUCES CENTRAL L5 PAIN —		
REP. EIL PRODUCES CENTRAL L5 PAIN AND DOES NOT WORSEN		

Neurological .. OK
Hip joints ... OK   S.I. OK
Conclusion: ~~Posture~~   Dysfunction   ~~Derangement~~
EXTENSION PRINCIPLE INITIALLY. CAN DERANGE.

PRINCIPLE OF TREATMENT   E.I.L. 10 X 6 AND POSTURE CORRECTION

patient *is* instructed in a self-treatment programme he is carefully warned *not to do* the exercises if they cause pain, thus defeating the purpose of the stretching.

If a patient receives manipulation in an attempt to lengthen contracted structures, minor trauma must follow and the dysfunction cycle will be perpetuated. If the patient receives only mobilisation procedures and does not perform exercises, the stretching that occurred during the ten minutes of treatment will be entirely lost by the contraction that is allowed to take place over the next twenty-three hours and fifty minutes, or whatever time period separates the treatment sessions. Even if exercises are given, no benefit will result unless the patient is instructed to move to the extreme range where some, but not great, discomfort or pain should be experienced. *If no strain pain is produced during the performance of exercises for the recovery of lost movement, the contracted soft tissues are not being stretched enough to enhance elongation of the shortened structures.* Furthermore, if the stretching procedures are not performed often enough, no benefit will result either. If the rest periods between the stretching procedures are too long, the length of time when no stretching takes place negates the effect of stretching.

We can have a significant influence on the remodelling of tissue expecially during the process of repair.[45]

In all dysfunction situations exercises for the restoration of movement and function must be performed about ten times per day from first thing in the morning to last thing at night. On each of the ten occasions a minimum of ten movements will be performed. In other words, the patient will perform one hundred stretches per day in groups of ten. The following instructions must be given to the patient:

— if the exercises do not produce some minor pain, the movement has not been performed far enough into the end range;
— the type of discomfort aimed at is not unlike the pain felt when bending the finger backwards beyond the normal position;
— the pain should have subsided within ten to twenty minutes after completion of the exercises;
— when pain produced *by* the stretching procedures lasts continuouly and is still evident the next day, overstretching — that is, too much stretching — has taken place; in this case the number of exercises in each sequence or the frequency of the sequences must be reduced.

It is accepted that due to circumstances many patients will be unable to strictly follow the recommended frequency of exercising. Where it is not possible to perform stretching as often as instructed, recovery of full function is likely to take a little longer.

During the course of one treatment session we should not use more than one new procedure; nor should that procedure, if it is a manipulative thrust technique, be performed more than once. Following the application of a new procedure or a manipulation we must wait, if necessary twenty-four hours, to assess the response of the patient.

Fig. 10:4. (opposite) *Clinical example of a typical patient with the dysfunction syndrome.*

TREATMENT OF EXTENSION DYSFUNCTION

By far the most common form of dysfunction is that involving loss of extension. Having already explained and taught the postural requirements, we must now instruct the patient in the methods required to regain lost extension (Fig. 10:5). We must explain to him the reasons for the need to recover the extension movement. The patient must realise that without an adequate range of extension it is not possible to sit with a lordosis, even when a lumbar support is used. For some patients it is imperative that the range of extension be improved, otherwise they will be unable to sit correctly. It is my experience that, following adequate explanation, patients will co-operate with the treatment and work hard at their recovery. They will perform exercises that cause discomfort or even pain, as long as they understand the reasons for doing so.

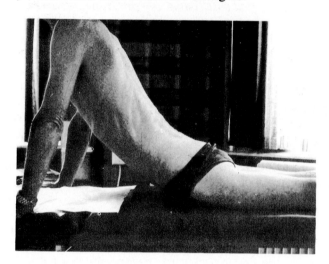

Fig. 10:5.
Recovery of loss of extension, using the procedure of extension in lying.

Exercises

In order to systematically stretch the lumbar spine in extension, I have adopted a system in which the patient is able to use gravity and his own body weight to apply enough force for adequate passive stretching of the joints of the lumbar spine. This procedure, a modified press-up exercise, is extension in lying (**Proc. 8:3**)*. If with this exercise the desired result is not obtained quickly enough or if progress ceases, extension in lying with belt fixation (**Proc. 8:4**) must be commenced.

If due to circumstances it is absolutely impossible to perform extension exercises in lying, extension in standing (**Proc. 8:6**) must be performed instead. But it must be emphasised that a far better extension stretch is obtained with extension exercises in lying (**Proc. 8:3 and 8:4**).

---

* Procedures will be referred to as follows:
(**Proc. 8:3**) means Chapter 8; Procedure 3.

The patient should be instructed to perform the exercise ten times on each occasion, and to repeat the series ten times a day at intervals of approximately two hours. It is most important to ensure that stretching occurs very regularly and the patient does not let more than two to three hours pass by without doing so.

The exercise routine should result in an increase of localised central back pain which subsides within ten to twenty minutes. The patient should also develop some new pains higher up in the spine and across the shoulders. These are normally the result of performing new exercises and holding a new posture. It is necessary to explain that the combination of the new posture and exercises will result in discomfort felt in other places; that this new aching is unavoidable and indeed necessary, but will pass after a week or so. Patients who do not complain of these transitional pains are probably not exercising adequately.

Irrespective of the category in which they may fall, all patients should be warned of the significance of producing peripheral pain. If exercises are found to produce peripheral pain, the patient should stop and wait until the next treatment when further advice should be sought.

The loss of function in patients in this group is usually resolved gradually over a period of about four to six weeks. After this period the patient may reduce the number of times the exercises are performed to four sessions per day, maintaining the number of ten repetitions at each session. I instruct my extension dysfunction patients that they should continue the programme and perform ten exercises twice daily for the rest of their lives.

Often it is desirable to keep some record of progress and the therapist may choose to take photographs to evaluate the improvement in the lumbar extension curve. The improvement is most evident in the first week, and therefore the first photographs should be taken on the first day prior to the commencement of the self-treatment programme.

Special techniques

As soon as progress slows down or ceases it is time to add mobilisation techniques (**Proc. 8:7 and 8:9**). If after three to four mobilisation treatments no change is evident, the patient should be manipulated (**Proc. 8:8 and 8:10**). Special techniques of mobilisation and manipulation are indicated, when the patient is unable to fully restore lumbar extension himself. These procedures may ensure full recovery of extension provided the extension exercises in lying (**Proc. 8:3 and 8:4**) are continued as well.

TREATMENT OF FLEXION DYSFUNCTION

Loss of flexion is the second most common movement loss in the lumbar spine (Fig. 10:6). It manifests itself in several ways, which interfere with either the amount of available flexion or the pathway taken to achieve flexion. This type of dysfunction is commonly seen in patients with an accentuated lordosis.

Patients with significant flexion dysfunction are usually unable to sit slouched with a convex lumbar spine. When giving postural instructions to these patients, we must explain that once sitting relaxed they place the lumbar spine on full stretch much sooner than patients with a normal flexion excursion.

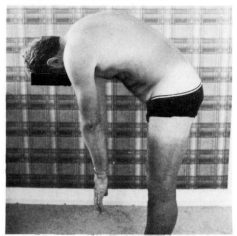

Fig. 10:6.
Recovery of loss of flexion, using the procedure of flexion in standing.

Recovery of pure flexion loss

To regain flexion we must, just as in the case of extension dysfunction, explain to the patient the purpose of performing exercises. Again, we must stress the necessity of causing a moderate degree of discomfort or pain with the exercises. Pain produced by stretching of contracted structures involved in the loss of flexion should be felt across the low back. Often it resembles the pain of which the patient originally complained, and as in the recovery of extension it should be shortlived.

Exercises

Recovery of pure flexion is commenced with exercises. The patient must perform flexion in lying (**Proc. 8:13**). This exercise should be performed ten times about every two hours. As said before, frequency and regularity of exercising are important factors in the treatment of dysfunction. When five to six days have passed the patient will describe that the knees can be bent fully onto the chest. All flexion that can possibly be restored in this position is now recovered, and the exercise no longer produces pain. In order to apply full passive stretch to regain the last few degrees of lumbar flexion it is necessary to perform flexion in standing (**Proc. 8:14**).

Up till now flexion has been performed in lying (**Proc. 8:13**) with elimination of gravitational forces. This rarely makes the patient significantly worse. In flexion in standing (**Proc. 8:14**) gravitational stresses are added.

When applied to dysfunction resulting from *recent* derangement, flexion in standing (**Proc. 8:14**) may sometimes exacerbate the condition. Therefore, when commencing flexion in standing (**Proc. 8:14**) the patient should reduce the number of exercises performed at each session as well as the frequency of the sessions per day — for example, five to six repetitions of the exercise should be done five to six times per day. This way there is little risk of exacerbation, and after four to five days the patient may progress to a full programme. Eventually the patient will recover his flexion and will almost reach the ground before any strain pain is felt. No discomfort should be experienced on returning to the erect position.

Special techniques

If full flexion cannot be restored by the patient's own efforts, the application of special procedures may be indicated, such as rotation mobilisation and manipulation in flexion (**Proc. 8:11 and 8:12**).

Occasionally, a patient with the derangement syndrome will mistakenly be placed in the dysfunction category. If this occurs the flexion procedures may immediately and significantly worsen the symptoms, and in this way the true nature of the condition will be revealed. Consequently, the treatment programme must be altered appropriately.

N.B. Remember that the recovery of function in flexion following recent derangement, is hazardous. Extension in lying (**Proc. 8:3**) should always follow flexion movements in order that any posterior disturbance is corrected immediately.

Treatment of flexion with deviation

There are two common types of deviation in flexion resulting from dysfunction. The first one occurs in the patient who is unable to reach full flexion via the normal sagittal pathway, no matter how hard he tries. Due to adaptively shortened structures within the intervertebral segment he is forced to deviate to one side during flexion.

Treatment for this type of flexion loss may follow the course recommended for recovery of pure flexion loss. Thus, treatment commences with flexion in lying (**Proc. 8:13**). Provided the initial twenty-four hour period of flexion in lying (**Proc. 8:13**) has not caused a *lasting* increase or peripheralisation of pain, the use of flexion in step standing (**Proc. 8:15**) is indicated at an early stage of treatment to correct the deviation in flexion. This is later followed by flexion in standing (**Proc. 8:14**) to ensure recovery of full flexion movement. When commencing flexion in step standing (**Proc. 8:15**) the same precautions should be taken as discussed previously (that is, when commencing flexion in standing (**Proc. 8:14**) in treatment recommended for recovery of pure flexion).

If the initial twenty-four hour period of flexion in lying (**Proc. 8:13**) causes a lasting increase or peripheralisation of symptoms, our diagnosis is incorrect and the most likely reason for the deviation is internal derangement of a lumbar disc. Consequently, we must alter our treatment approach.

The second type of deviation in flexion resulting from dysfunction is caused by an adherent nerve root, and its treatment will be discussed in conjunction with the treatment of sciatica.

TREATMENT OF SIDE GLIDING DYSFUNCTION — CORRECTION OF SECONDARY LATERAL SHIFT

Having observed thousands of lumbar spines it has become clear to me that asymmetry is the 'norm' and symmetry is almost atypical. Therefore, when examining dysfunction patients it is important to realise that many exhibit a minor scoliosis or lateral shift, the direction of which is sometimes extremely difficult to determine. With careful observation it can be seen that the top half of the patient's body is not correctly related to the bottom half, and the patient has shifted laterally about the lumbar area (Fig. 10:7). The anomalies include a number of lateral shifts now dysfunctional in character. These lateral shifts are referred to as secondary whereas those caused by derangement are primary.

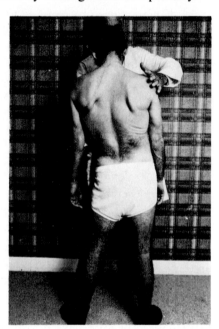

Fig. 10:7.
Recovery of loss of side gliding,
teaching the procedure of self-
correction of secondary lateral shift.

As discussed previously, we must determine whether the lateral shift is relevant to the present symptoms or is merely a congenital or developmental anomaly. If side gliding produces pain there is likely to be adaptive shortening within or about the disc and recovery of the side gliding movement must be attempted. As it is not easy to apply overpressure in the side gliding exercise, it may be difficult to recover this movement.

The patient must be fully instructed in self-correction of lateral shift (**Proc. 8:17**). He should perform the procedure ten times per day, at each session moving ten times into the overcorrected position. The last movement should be held firmly for about thirty to forty seconds. The patient should also be encouraged to stand in the overcorrected position whenever an opportunity arises during the day. If by the end of the first week pain produced by lateral shift correction is much less, the procedure will most likely have the desired result and must be continued for about three to four weeks in an attempt to restore full function. But if no change is evident after one week, there is little hope of improving this aspect of dysfunction.

TYPICAL TREATMENT PROGRESSION — THE DYSFUNCTION SYNDROME

Day one

— Assessment and conclusion/diagnosis.
— Explanation of the cause of dysfunction and the treatment approach.
— Postural correction and instructions, especially regarding sitting; demonstrate the use of a lumbar support.
— Commence with exercises to recover function — that is, extension in lying, flexion in lying, or side gliding in standing, whatever procedure is indicated.
— Emphasise the need to experience some discomfort during the exercises, and the importance of frequent exercising during the day.
— If flexion in lying is recommended, we must warn to stop exercising if the symptoms quickly worsen. We may have overlooked derangement, or commenced the procedure too early following recent derangement.
— Always follow flexion exercises with some extension.

Day two

— Confirm diagnosis.
— Check postural correction.
— Completely repeat'postural correction and instructions.
— Check exercises. If improving nothing should be changed.
— If not improving, ensure that exercises are performed *far enough* into end range, maintained *long enough* during the last three repetitions, and performed *often enough* during the day.
— Warn for 'new pains'.

Day three

— Check posture and exercises.
— If no improvement, commence mobilisation procedures. Several mobilisation treatments may be required.
— Patient must continue the self-treatment exercises as directed.

Day four and five

— Check exercises and progress.
— If in treatment for flexion dysfunction no further progress is possible with flexion in lying, change to flexion in standing, possibly flexion in step standing.
— Take necessary precautions when starting flexion in standing.
— Ensure that patient has 'new pains'.

Further treatments

— I prefer to see patients in this category three or four days in succession. If progress is adequate and the patient understands the self-treatment programme, treatment may change to alternate days and later to twice per week if required.
— It usually takes ten to twelve treatments, spread over four to six weeks, to successfully treat dysfunction.
— If towards the middle of the treatment period the patient ceases to improve and especially if the remaining pain is unilateral, then a rotation manipulation may be required. This may have to be repeated two or three times and should be combined with mobilising and exercising procedures already being applied.
— Before discharge prophylaxis must be discussed in detail.

CHAPTER 11

The Derangement Syndrome

Of all mechanical low back problems that are encountered in general medical practise, mechanical derangement of the intervertebral disc is potentially the most disabling. It is my belief that in the lumbar spine, if in no other area, disturbance of the intervertebral disc mechanism is responsible for the production of symptoms in as many as ninety-five percent of our patients. Twenty-five years of clinical observation and treatment of lumbar conditions have convinced me that certain phenomena and the various movements which affect them, can occur only because of the hydrostatic properties invested in the intervertebral disc.

For thirty years Cyriax[24] has attributed lumbar pain to internal derangement of the intervertebral disc mechanism. He has outlined the cause of lumbago, and proposed that pain of a slow onset is likely to be produced by a nuclear protrusion while that of a sudden onset is caused by a displaced annular fragment. Although at present we are unable to prove either of these hypotheses, I support his general view that the disc is the cause of much lumbar pain; but I cannot believe that slow and sudden onsets of pain can be so clearly separated and ascribed to different structures within the same disc.

Various authorities describe phenomena — observed clinically, at surgery, and in cadaveric experiments — that indicate aberrant behaviour of structures within the disc complex. Mathews[37] reports that a small bulge of a lumbar disc may cause pain in the back and asymmetry of the involved intervertebral articulation, leading to scoliosis and asymmetrical limitation of movement of the lumbar spine. Nachemson[38] describes bulging of the annulus under loading conditions, and increased bulging with movements of the spinal column. Vernon-Roberts[23] states that during surgical explorations of disc prolapses some protrusions were seen to alternately protrude into the spinal canal and retreat into the disc substance, depending on the type of movement the lumbar spine was subjected to. Moreover, according to Mathews[37] myelograms were seen to be positive only when taken with patients in the painful position, a further indication of the relationship between disc bulge and increased pain on movements. Thus, it is evident that *minor disc bulging may cause deformity and limitation of movement,* and that *certain movements of the spinal column increase the bulge while others may reduce it.*

The ability of the nucleus to move anteriorly in extension, posteriorly in flexion and laterally in lateral flexion[13, 21] depends very much on the integrity of the annular wall, for it has been found that the position of the nuclear fluids can be affected by movement only as long as the hydrostatic mechanism is intact. Park[27] has shown that in frank nuclear protrusions the opaque medium, injected in the disc, remains contained in a localised area irrespective of the position of the spine. Once nuclear material has escaped through the annular wall, the hydrostatic mechanism is no longer intact and internal derangement of the disc cannot be reduced significantly by movements of the spinal column. On the other hand, movements of the spinal column can be utilised to reverse internal derangement of the disc as long as the integrity of the disc wall is maintained.

In conclusion, we have now ample evidence that movements of the spinal column effect the position of the nucleus within the disc under certain circumstances; and there is enough proof to incriminate the disc as the cause of the deformities so often encountered in patients with low back pain, particularly in the acute stages. It cannot be disputed that certain movements and positions lead to the development of these deformities; and, likewise, that other movements and positions can be utilised to reduce these deformities.

Many doctors are still under the impression that the pain of 'lumbago' necessarily has an inflammatory component. If this were true, reduction of derangement would never provide immediate and lasting relief from pain as often occurs.

It must be well understood that pain resulting from inflammation has a chemical origin, and will only be present as long as there is enough chemical irritation of the free nerve endings. Inflammatory pain cannot possibly on one movement appear in the buttock, and on another movement disappear from the buttock and appear in the midline of the back. Pain that changes site with movement must result from mechanical deformation — that is, before movement took place different structures or different parts of the same structure were subjected to mechanical deformation than during or after movement. The actual cause of the mechanical deformation — the structure producing it — has changed its position or shape during the movement.

DEFINITION

I would define derangement as the situation in which the normal resting position of the articular surfaces of two adjacent vertebrae is disturbed as a result of a change in the position of the fluid nucleus between these surfaces. The alteration in the position of the nucleus may also disturb annular material. This change within the joint will affect the ability of the joint surfaces to move in their normal relative pathways and departures from these pathways are frequently seen. In some patients movements may only be reduced but in others they will be lost entirely. Usually, the movement involved is either flexion or extension and often a loss of side gliding can be seen in conjunction.

In addition to causing losses of movement in the lumbar segments, derangement of the disc can cause the deformities of kyphosis and scoliosis.

Acute lumbar kyphosis

The stresses most likely to cause an acute lumbar kyphosis are sustained flexion stresses such as those applied during gardening and in sitting. Prolonged maintenance of flexed positions and frequent repetition of movements in flexion, especially when extension is never fully recovered, may both lead to excessive accumulation of the fluid nucleus in the posterior compartment between the vertebral bodies. Once this accumulation is great enough it may become a blockage and prevent the erect position from being obtained. Any attempt by the patient to straighten up quickly leads to significant pain, as the compressive forces create bulging of the posterior longitudinal ligament and annulus which are now under extreme tangential stress. The patient must return to the flexed position in order to reduce the intensity of the pain. We now have an acute lumbar kyphosis. The patient is not held in this position by muscle spasm.[24]

In acute lumbar kyphosis the incidence of sciatica is relatively low. The postero-central disc bulging which causes the kyphosis, must move laterally before it can reach the nerve root. Once it has moved laterally the patient will develop a scoliosis. Consequently, most patients with sciatica have some degree of lateral shift or scoliosis.

Acute lumbar scoliosis

It appears reasonable to suggest that the posterior longitudinal ligament may prevent postero-central disturbances in the disc wall. However, sooner or later asymmetrical stresses will force the fluid nucleus laterally where the outer annulus will distend at its weakest point. There is greater elasticity and decreased resistance to distention at the posterior surface of the disc, especially where the larger radius curve meets the smaller one.[39] Here the annulus is narrowest and less firmly attached to the bone, and is not reinforced by the posterior longitudinal ligament. Therefore, bulging of the annulus is more likely to occur at this point than anywhere else.

To recapitulate, a patient with lumbago may obtain the deformity of kyphosis by a posterior movement of the nucleus. Should this symmetrical posterior accumulation become asymmetrical and move to a more postero-lateral position within the intervertebral compartment, the patient is likely to develop sciatica and will acquire the deformity of scoliosis. Thus, a patient with lumbar kyphosis and low back pain merely has to move to one side or other to run the risk of changing his deformity to a scoliosis. For example, a side bending or torsion movement to the left will cause the nucleus to move to the right; with sufficient accumulation of nuclear material on the right side the patient will have difficulting in obtaining the erect posture and will develop a lateral shift to the left.

I have recorded the progression from acute kyphosis to acute scoliosis many times clinically. During the development of my treatment methods I discovered that it is possible to induce a scoliosis in a patient presenting with an acute kyphosis and then to reduce it, provided the appropriate procedure is applied in time.

History

Patients with low back pain caused by derangement are commonly between twenty and fifty-five years of age. From that time on the incidence of the derangement syndrome reduces gradually as degenerative processes develop and progress. Men appear to be affected by derangement more often than women.[10, 12]

Low back pain is notorious for its recurrent nature. It is suggested that ninety percent of people with low back pain will have recurrent problems.[40] I estimate that sixty-two of every hundred patients will become recurrent. The majority of patients with recurrent problems occur in the derangement syndrome.

Derangement of the lumbar intervertebral disc may arise from a single severe strain,[9] a less severe strain applied more frequently, or a sustained flexion strain. The latter is most common and occurs in people who have a sedentary occupation or work in stooped positions. Sustained flexion positions force the nucleus to the extreme within its cavity and, as a result of time, posterior accumulation of nuclear material beyond the normal limit may prevent the attainment of movements and positions opposite to the sustained flexed position. The length of time that a particular position has been held often determines the degree of derangement.

When movements are constantly varied in direction the fluid nucleus never occupies a fixed position for any length of time and continuously alters its silhouette. Provided movements do not cause excessive strain and are not repeated too regularly, accumulation of nuclear material will not occur. Likewise, the simple action of flexion — that is, bending forwards once without placing great strains on the lumbar spine and without having been in sustained flexion prior to bending — is unlikely to cause an episode of low back pain. Many patients blame the simple forward bending movement for the onset of their pain, but on close questioning there has usually been a position or an activity involving prolonged flexion preceding the onset of pain. Let me further illustrate this.

Clinical examples:

A lady states that her low back pain came on as she merely stooped to pick up a button. However, further questioning reveals that she had been in sustained flexion — sitting in front of her sewing machine — for some time immediately prior to bending down.

Similarly, the man who removed his golf clubs from the rear compartment of his car did not develop pain because he suddenly flexed. He had been driving his car and sat in flexion for some time before he got out of the car and bent over to pick up his golf clubs. It is unlikely that he straightened up fully after leaving the car, and the additional flexion to lift his golf clubs from the car surely raised the intradiscal pressure in a joint that was already under considerable stress. These are typical examples of derangement with a rapid onset.

Now an example of derangement with a slow onset. A patient worked in the garden at the beginning of spring. It was some time since he had any exercise. He spent the entire afternoon digging and noticed that a mild ache developed in his low back. As the day wore on he had some difficulty in rising from the stooped position. After he stopped working he had a hot bath and felt a little easier, sat down for his evening meal, read the newspaper and watched television for a while. He had great difficulty rising from his chair and never really obtained the upright position before he went to bed. He had a very disturbed night, and could only lie curled up on his right side. When he awoke the next morning he could hardly get up from his bed and had difficulty walking. By this time he felt severe low back pain and was tilted to one side as well as forwards.

Variations on similar themes are described every day and on most occasions flexion stress is the basic cause of derangement. When pure flexion strains are described the pain tends to be central or bilateral with symmetrical distribution. But if an asymmetrical movement involving flexion and rotation or side bending is the causative factor, the site of pain tends to become unilateral.

It is interesting to note that in the majority of patients presenting with derangement, the time of onset is before midday. Due to the nocturnal imbibition of the disc the volume of intradiscal fluid is increased which allows for greater nuclear excursion and distortion whenever stresses are placed on the disc. I believe that during the first five to six hours after rising in the morning the risks of incurring derangement are greatest.

One of the most important questions when taking the history of patients with low back pain is that regarding the intermittency or constancy of the pain. *Mechanical deformation resulting from postural stresses or dysfunction always causes intermittent pain. Mechanical deformation due to derangement, by its very nature and definition, nearly always causes constant pain.* In derangement the adjacent joint surfaces are disturbed from their normal position so that some of the structures within and around the involved joint are under constant stress. These will be a source of constant pain until the stress is removed either by reduction of the derangement or by adaptive lengthening. Thus, whenever a patient describes constant pain and the pain is constant indeed, — that is, there is no time in the day when pain is not present — he is almost certain to have a derangement. Of course, this influences very much the treatment he will receive and the direction in which movement procedures must be applied.

While the presence of constant pain strongly suggests derangement, not all patients with derangement have constant pain. There is a group of patients who state that they have no pain at all as long as they are on the move, but once they maintain a position, pain will be felt after a few minutes. Movement and a change of position brings about a short-lived respite from pain, which is soon felt again and necessitates a further change of position. The temporary relief is caused by a reduction of stress on the structures presently causing pain, but at the same time other structures are placed under stress and rapidly become painful.

There are also patients in whom, during the course of the day and depending on their activities, minor derangements are alternatively produced and reduced spontaneously. In these patients the intermittent pain is caused by intermittent derangements which are self-reducing.

In the derangement syndrome the pain will be made worse under certain circumstances. Usually these circumstances involve positions rather than movements. The majority of patients will experience an increase of pain in flexed positions, and when a scoliosis or lateral shift is present extension will cause an increase in pain as well as flexion.

Sitting is the most common aggravating factor for all low back pain syndromes. Rising from sitting increases pain in derangement syndrome only.

When patients describe a history in which both walking and sitting enhance pain, they are likely to exhibit a lateral shift.[10] In the presence of a lateral shift any attempt to extend the lumbar spine will cause or increase pain, and walking produces enough extension to enhance pain.

In general, if the derangement is small patients feel better when on the move and worse when at rest. However, if the derangement is large and causes significant deformity patients usually feel better when lying down.

Patients with derangement often have difficulty in finding a comfortable sleeping position. They cannot lie supine with the legs out straight because the available range of extension is inadequate. Prone lying is prevented for the same reason. The only position in which some comfort can be derived is by lying supine with the knees flexed or on the side with the knees bent up, both positions placing the lumbar spine in flexion. Following either of these, patients have considerable difficulty arising in the morning. In sub-acute patients extension remains blocked for up to an hour and is only gradually regained if at all. In acute patients the pain is so severe that they prefer to return to bed, where they resume the flexed position which relieves their pain for the present time but perpetuates their problem.

In North America, where the flexion therapy philosophy is strongest, patients with acute low back pain are advised to rest in flexed positions, and extraordinary measures are taken to ensure the maintenance of flexion while in bed. However, on questioning patients with derangement they almost universally complain that, after sleeping in such a position, they have difficulty on rising from lying and their pain is markedly increased when coming to the erect position. Pain experienced first thing in the morning when getting up is frequently the result of the overnight posture of the patient. If the spine is held in such a position during the night that the nucleus accumulates posteriorly, it is extremely difficult and painful to reduce this derangement rapidly. Sometimes several hours must pass before reduction can be achieved. The same mechanism causes the increase of pain felt when the patient with posterior derangement rises from sitting to standing.

Examination

On examination, the patient with derangement *often* exhibits a deformity. Commonly seen deformities are the flattened lumbar spine or lumbar kyphosis,

(Fig. 11:1) and the lateral shift or lumbar scoliosis (Fig. 11:2). There is *always* loss of movement and function, (Fig. 11:3) and in contrast to dysfunction the movement loss is nearly always asymmetrical. In addition, there may be a departure from the normal pathway of movement (Fig. 11:3). In derangement this departure may be a deviation to the right or left of the sagittal plane. I believe this pathway is determined by the position of the disturbance in the nucleus/annulus complex. Should the nucleus be displaced abnormally to the right of the midline, the deviation will occur to the left.

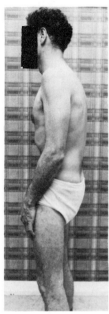
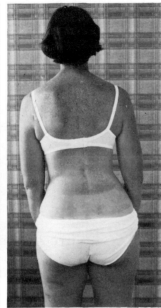
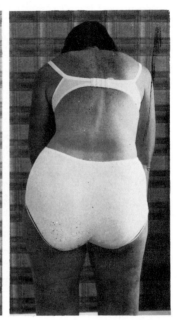

Fig. 11:1.	Fig. 11:2.	Fig. 11:3.
Deformity of kyphosis.	*Deformity of scoliosis.*	*Deviation in flexion.*

Cyriax[24] already disposed of the misconception that spasm of the extensor muscles in the back is responsible for the production of an acute lumbar kyphosis. I join him in this view and would like to add than an acute lumbar scoliosis is not caused by muscle spasm, neither is a departure from the normal pathway of movement. The position of the nucleus within the disc predetermines the alignment of the joint surfaces between two adjacent vertebral bodies, and therefore dictates the pathway to be followed during movement and the position to be maintained during rest.

The test movements

The test movements are performed to determine the nature of the presenting syndrome — that is, dysfunction or derangement — and the severity of the condition. In derangement there is rarely, if ever, any difficulty in producing or increasing the symptoms, and often centralisation can be observed as well. *Centralisation of symptoms occurs only in the derangement syndrome.*

The test movements are designed to reveal the presence of derangement. They alternately increase and decrease the disturbance by changing the position of the nucleus within the intervertebral disc and altering the stresses on the surrounding annulus and posterior longitudinal ligament. When the history suggests that a potentially disabling situation is present, it is *not desirable to develop the flexion testing procedures* to the bitter end. In these cases flexion in standing is often too painful to be repeated, and each successive movement may increase or peripheralise the pain. Sometimes repeated flexion in lying has the same effect. In derangement, the increase or peripheralisation of pain with each repeated movement indicates a rapidly increasing derangement. When this occurs we should not insist on completing the recommended number of test movements.

When the test movements affect pain it is important to state clearly whether pain is *produced or increased*. The former indicates that there was no pain before the test movements were performed and the test movements actually produced pain. The latter means that pain, present before the performance of test movements, has increased as a result of them. It is imperative that we establish the existing pain state before commencing the test movements in order to be able to assess the effects of these test movements on pain.

If a patient with derangement describes changes in the pain pattern following the test movements, there should also be observable changes in range of movement and deformity. In other words, a patient who describes a significant increase in pain should exhibit an increase in the mechanical blockage of movement and deformity — that is, a reduction of movement range and an increase of deformity; and the patient who describes a reduction in pain must simultaneously exhibit an increase in range of movement and a reduction of deformity.

In derangement the repetition of the test movements can have a rapid effect on the condition and the patient may improve or worsen in a matter of minutes depending on the direction in which the movements are performed. When the test movements are repeated in the direction which increases the accumulation of nuclear material, pain will increase with each successive movement and after the treatment the patient may remain significantly worse as a result of increased derangement. The opposite applies when the test movements are repeated in the direction which reduces the derangement. In this case the patient improves with each successive movement and remains improved subsequently. In general, *rapid and lasting changes in the condition as a result of the test movements are an indication of derangement.*

If the annular wall is breached, we cannot influence the position of the nucleus with normal movements of the spine. This situation appears clinically in the patient with sciatica who has constant pain and cannot find relief by either positioning or movement. Most of the test movements can be seen to enhance his leg pain and no test movement will reduce it. Thus, the performance of the test movements clarifies the severity of the derangement situation.

Fig. 11:4. (opposite) *Clinical example of a typical patient with the derangement syndrome.*

LUMBAR SPINE ASSESSMENT

Date.......... 20 APRIL 1980

Name.......... JOHN SMITH

Address........... CHATSWORTH ROAD

SILVERSTREAM

Date of birth...... 20 APRIL 1931

Occupation ...... UNEMPLOYED

HISTORY

Symptoms now ...... PAIN (R) L4.5 INTO (R) BUTTOCK

...... AND POSTERIOR THIGH

at onset......... CENTRE AND (R) L5

Present for......... 12 DAYS

Commenced as a result of...... RISING FROM SITTING

No apparent reason. ☐

Constant/~~Intermittent~~. ✓

When worse — bending, ✓ sitting or rising from, ✓ PROLONGED standing, ✓ walking, lying. ✓ SUPINE

Other ......

When better — bending, sitting or rising from, standing, walking, ✓ lying. ✓

Other ...... MOVING PRONE

Disturbed sleep — Yes ~~No~~ ON TURNING Cough/sneeze +ve ~~-ve~~

Previous history...... 3 X IN PAST 5 YEARS (ACUTE) 5 – 6 MINOR.

and treatment...... BED REST – BRACE – CHIROPRACTIC

X-Rays ...... NO ABNORMALITIES DETECTED

General health ...... OK   Meds/Steroids ...... NO

Recent surgery ...... NO   Accident...... NO

Gait ...... OK   Bladder ...... OK

EXAMINATION

Posture sitting ...... POOR   Lordosis reduced/~~accentuated~~......

Posture standing......... NOT BAD   Leg length ...... OK

Lateral shift (R) or (L) or ~~nil~~

MOVEMENT LOSS

Flexion: Major. ~~Moderate.~~ ~~Minimal.~~ Deviation (R) or (L)......

Extension: ~~Major.~~ Moderate. ~~Minimal.~~ Deviation (R) or (L)......

Side Gliding: (R) or ~~(L)~~ ......

TEST MOVEMENTS

FIS. PRODUCES BUTTOCK PAIN   SGIS (R) ...... NO CHANGE

REP. FIS " THIGH PAIN AND WORSENS   SGIS (L) ...... ↑ BUTTOCK PAIN

EIS ↑ PAIN (R)L5 ↓ BUTTOCK   REP. SGIS (R) ...... NO CHANGE

REP. EIS ↑ " " ABOLISHED BUTTOCK PAIN   REP. SGIS (L) ...... ↗ BUTTOCK PAIN

FIL PRODUCES BUTTOCK PAIN

REP. FIL WORSENS BUTTOCK PAIN

EIL PRODUCES PAIN ACROSS L5. NO BUTTOCK OR THIGH PAIN

REP. EIL CENTRALISES PAIN AT (R) L5. BUT DOES NOT ABOLISH

Neurological ...... OK

Hip joints...... OK   S.I. OK

Conclusion: ~~Posture~~ ~~Dysfunction~~ Derangement 4

PRINCIPLE OF TREATMENT

SHIFT CORRECTION AND EXTENSION PRINCIPLE AND POSTURE CORRECTION. PROBABLY UNDERLYING DYSFUNCTION.

Clinical examples:

Let us now look at the example of a typical patient with derangement (Fig. 11:4). He states that he has constant pain, but is better on the move than in any of the positions. Walking and lying prone also improve the symptoms. The test movements clearly show increase and peripheralisation of pain on the flexion movements, and centralisation of symptoms occurs during extension. This patient will benefit from the extension principle, and hopefully his constant pain will become intermittent with the regular use of extension procedures.

A few more examples will demonstrate the importance of centralisation of symptoms during test movements and treatment of the patient with derangement.

A patient complains of pain extending evenly across the low back to about ten centimeters on either side of the midline. This pain has been present for some months and is usually worse when working in flexed positions or sitting for a while. The test movements reveal that on repeated flexion the pain spreads further across the low back, and on repeated extension the pain increases but moves towards the midline. Further extension movements cause a reduction in intensity of that pain. Extension clearly is the movement that reduces the derangement and should be used in the treatment. If extension is continued and performed regularly over the next twenty-four hours, the pain should become less and less and should be under control within that time period.

A young woman complains of pain across the low back and aching into both buttocks and thighs. She states that the pain increases in the back during prolonged standing — extension — and moves into buttocks and thighs during walking — increased extension. — However, on sitting down — flexion — the pain leaves the legs and is felt only in the back, and after ten minutes of sitting — sustained flexion — it has subsided completely. Again the centralisation phenomenon shows us that in this case extension movements are increasing the derangement and therefore should be avoided. On the other hand, flexion is reducing the derangement and is the correct principle of treatment for this patient.

Straight-leg-raising

Patients with sciatica, especially those who also exhibit a deformity of scoliosis and have constant pain, will have a limitation of straight-leg-raising on the side of the sciatica. Furthermore, straight-leg-raising will be limited in patients who are in the acute stage of a severe derangement condition. In these patients all movements aggravate the symptoms, and often relief is obtained only when lying in bed and keeping as still as possible.

Let us examine the relevance of straight-leg-raising, performed as an objective testing procedure. When a limitation of straight-leg-raising is found, there is always a restriction of flexion in standing as well. It is virtually impossible to have a limitation of straight-leg-raising and be able to flex pelvis and lumbar spine in a normal fashion. Some patients appear to have full flexion in standing, but on close observation they can be seen to deviate in flexion and to move in an arc to one side or other rather than in the sagittal plane. In patients with sciatica and root entrapment, deviation occurs always to the side of referred pain as this is the side where nerve root impingement takes place. The patients are unable to control the deviation in flexion themselves.

There is nothing that can be elicited by straight-leg-raising tests, that is not evident in careful observation of flexion in standing. When there is increased tension of the nerve root the straight-leg-raising limitation appears to occur much sooner than does the restriction of flexion in standing. This is because the straight-leg-raising test is performed in supine lying, and in this position deviation of the spine is difficult. There only appears to be a better range of flexion in standing, because deviation of the spine allows more flexion towards the side of root tension. If the deviation is prevented from occurring by holding the patient in the sagittal plane, an immediate reduction in the flexion range becomes apparent. This reduction in the range of flexion will now coincide with the degree of straight-leg-raising.

Another test may help to understand the mechanism involved in restriction of straight-leg-raising. When performing straight-leg-raising, do not stop the movement immediately when sciatica is produced or increased. Instead, continue to raise the leg firmly but slowly, and at the same time observe the pelvis. At first it can be seen to rotate to the opposite side, then it tilts backwards while the lumbar spine flattens and commences to flex. This is merely an inverted version of the deviation of flexion in standing.

Straight-leg-raising is an extremely unreliable test and as an objective tool only of use in determining the progress of patients with entrapment.

TREATMENT OF THE DERANGEMENT SYNDROME

Of all patients with low back pain those having derangement of the intervertebral disc are the most interesting and rewarding to treat. As in dysfunction, it is essential in derangement that from the very first treatment correction of the sitting posture be achieved, but in the early and acute stages of derangement emphasis is placed on the *maintenance of lordosis* rather than the obtaining of the correct posture. Failure in this respect means failure of what otherwise might be a successful reduction of the derangement. So often it occurs that a patient describes a significant relief from pain and is visibly improved immediately following treatment, but later that same day after sitting for some time he is unable to straighten up on rising from sitting and the symptoms have returned just as they were before treatment. Usually the patient clearly understands the dangers of bending and stooping and carefully avoids these movements. *But the hidden dangers of sustained flexion incurred in the sitting position is rarely recognised by patient or therapist.*

Two of every three patients with low back pain have symptoms commencing for no apparent reason.[10] Where there is no recognisable precipitating strain in the production of mechanical back pain, we must assume that the symptoms commenced as a result of the patient's normal daily pursuits. In other words, in the course of every day living the patient has performed a series of movements or adopted certain positions which have led to mechanical derangement within the lumbar spine. I believe that it is possible to equip the patient with the necessary information and instruct him in the methods required to reverse the mechanical disturbances he unwittingly created and to prevent further episodes of low back pain. This can be achieved if instructions and explanations are given in an adequate but simple manner.

If the patient adopted a position or performed a movement that damaged the disc mechanism, utilisation of the patient's movements can reverse that derangement if we understand the mechanism involved.

Where time is a crucial factor in the production of derangement, it must be utilised to its advantage in the reduction of the same. For example, if pain is stated to arise commonly after half an hour of sitting and is caused by derangement, it is unlikely to appear clinically after only two minutes of flexion; and if it takes thirty minutes to produce pain clinically it is unlikely to disappear in two minutes. Throughout the treatment of derangement ample time must be allowed for the distorted nucleus to alter its silhouette and for reversal of the flow of displaced nuclear gel within the disc. In the reduction of derangement, time is obtained by sustaining positions or repeating movements.

During the course of one treatment session we should not use more than one new procedure; nor should that procedure, if it is a manipulative thrust technique, be performed more than once. Following the application of a new procedure or a manipulation we must wait, if necessary twenty-four hours, to assess the response of the patient.

There are several derangements which commonly occur in the lumbar spine. I realise that my classification of the derangements may oversimplify the true position, but for adequate explanation simplification is necessary. It must be appreciated that many variations of the derangements are possible and not all patients will neatly fit into the system.

Table of Derangements

Derangement One:

>Central or symmetrical pain across L4/5.
>Rarely buttock or thigh pain.
>No deformity.

Derangement Two:

>Central or symmetrical pain across L4/5.
>With or without buttock and/or thigh pain.
>With deformity of lumbar kyphosis.

Derangement Three:

>Unilateral or asymmetrical pain across L4/5.
>With or without buttock and/or thigh pain.
>No deformity.

Derangement Four:

>Unilateral or asymmetrical pain across L4/5.
>With or without buttock and/or thigh pain.
>With deformity of lumbar scoliosis.

Derangement Five:

>Unilateral or asymmetrical pain across L4/5.
>With or without buttock and/or thigh pain.
>With leg pain extending below the knee.
>No deformity.

Derangement Six:

>Unilateral or asymmetrical pain across L4/5.
>With or without buttock and/or thigh pain.
>With leg pain extending below the knee.
>With deformity of sciatic scoliosis.

Derangement Seven:

>Symmetrical or asymmetrical pain across L4/5.
>With or without buttock and/or thigh pain.
>With deformity of accentuated lumbar lordosis.

I believe that the postero-central and postero-lateral derangements (Derangements One to Six) are all progressions of the same disturbance within the intervertebral disc: commencing with Derangement One, which is the embryonic stage of posterior disc disturbance exhibiting central pain, each successive derangement shows peripheralisation of pain or development of deformity. *The principle aim of treatment is to centralise pain and reduce deformity in order to reverse all derangements to Derangement One. Patients with Derangement One are able to treat themselves.*

Under Derangement Seven fall the less common anterior and antero-lateral disc disturbances. The treatment follows a different course than for the posterior derangements, but also here the principle treatment aim is centralisation of pain and reduction of deformity.

In general, the treatment of derangement has four stages:

(1) reduction of derangement.
(2) maintenance of reduction.
(3) recovery of function.
(4) prevention of recurrence.

If possible, the first two stages will be achieved during the initial treatment session. Correction of sitting posture and instruction in a simple means of self-reduction in case of recurrence usually follow. Recovery of function will only be commenced once reduction of derangement has proven to be stable and the patient has been painfree for a few days. Before discharging the patient a full prophylactic programme is given. Self treatment is essential in prophylaxis.

Prophylaxis is impossible without self understanding.

CHAPTER 12

The Derangements and Their Treatment

DERANGEMENT ONE:

Central or symmetrical pain across L4/5.
Rarely buttock or thigh pain
No deformity

In Derangement One the disturbance within the disc is at a comparatively embryonic stage. Due to minor posterior migration of the nucleus and its invasion of a small radial fissure in the inner annulus, there is a minimal disturbance of disc material. This causes mechanical deformation of structures posteriorly within and about the disc, resulting in central or symmetrical low back pain. The accumulation of disc material also leads to a minor blockage in the affected joint preventing full extension, but the blockage is not enough to force the deformity of kyphosis upon the joint.

In patients with Derangement One the history, symptoms and signs are usually typical of the syndrome, and the test movements confirm the diagnosis of derangement. Because the disturbance within the joint is relatively small it responds well to the patients' own movements, and the majority of patients are able to reduce the derangement themselves by applying self-mobilising procedures. It is vitally important that all patients realise and experience the extent to which their own efforts of self-treatment contribute to the reduction of Derangement One. Therefore, *it is undesirable to use therapist-technique in the first twenty-four hours of treatment.*

Treatment

Reduction of derangement

The patient with Derangement One will require the application of the extension principle. He should start lying prone (**Proc. 8:1**)* for about five minutes, followed by lying prone in extension (**Proc. 8:2**) for another five minutes. He must then lie relaxed for a short while before commencing extension in lying (**Proc. 8:3**). This exercise, a modified press-up, should be done in groups of ten,

---

* Procedures will be referred to as follows:
  (**Proc. 8:1**) means (Chapter 8, Procedure 1).

and during the treatment session the groups are to be repeated five or six times with a rest period of about two minutes in between. During this time the patient should be questioned repeatedly to ensure that reduction of the derangement is taking place. At the completion of thirty or forty press-ups the range of extension should have improved significantly and the pain, if previously felt across the low back, should be localised more centrally. If before exercising the pain was already felt centrally, it should now be reduced in intensity. *When reduction is almost complete patients often state that the original pain is gone but a strain pain or stiffness is felt instead.* This can be achieved even during the first treatment session. No other procedure should be used if extension in lying **(Proc. 8:3)** culminates in centralisation or decrease in intensity of the presenting pain. If this occurs we can assume that there is a reduction in the magnitude of the derangement, and steps should now be taken to ensure that the reduction is maintained.

Maintenance of reduction

In order to maintain reduction of posterior derangement it is essential that *the lordosis is maintained at all times.* The patient should be instructed that at no time should he allow the lumbar spine to become flattened or convex. We must point out that if he is painfree in the prone lying position with the lumbar spine in extension, there is no reason why pain should arise in other positions such as sitting and standing or during movements and walking, provided that the same degree of extension is retained. If, with the lumbar spine in lordosis, the angle at which the affected joint is held prevents mechanical deformation, no pain will occur providing that angle is maintained.

Successful reduction of derangement will be shortlived if the patient subsequently sits without a lordosis. Sitting is usually the most troublesome position for patients with Derangement One. Bad sitting positions may cause and will definitely prolong symptoms of derangement. However, by maintaining the joints in the position of near maximum lordosis while sitting, the patient ensures that the fluid nucleus is held anteriorly. Of all the sitting positions the intradiscal pressure is at its lowest when sitting with a lordosis. Mechanical deformation will be minimal and the pain level will be greatly reduced in this position.

At this stage the patient should be shown *how to maintain* the lordosis in sitting. The slouch-overcorrect procedure should not be introduced as yet as it allows the patient to lose his lordosis. This procedure can be added once reduction of the derangement proves stable and the patient is ready for flexion procedures. In the early stages of treatment of Derangment One the patient is instructed to maintain the lordosis with his own muscular effort or with the use of a lumbar support. All patients with this type of derangement are advised to sit with a lumbar support, especially when driving the car or sitting in an easy chair.

Besides maintaining the lordosis the patient must be instructed to *repeat the exercises every waking hour for the next twenty-four hours.* Hourly repetition of the passively performed extension in lying (**Proc. 8:3**) ensures that no significant accumulation of nuclear material recurs in the posterior compartment of the joint. One group of ten repetitions of extension in lying (**Proc. 8:3**) is sufficient and it requires less than one minute to complete this. If circumstances prevent the performance of extension in lying (**Proc. 8:3**) it must be replaced by extension in standing (**Proc. 8:6**).

If following successful reduction, pain returns or increases to its former level at some time later in the day, it is likely that the patient has permitted some flexion to occur and has consequently lost the lordosis. He must take immediate steps to recover it, and usually one group of ten repetitions of extension in lying (**Proc. 8:3**) is sufficient but sometimes more may be required. Again, if circumstances prevent the performance of extension in lying (**Proc. 8:3**), extension in standing (**Proc. 8:6**) must be substituted.

Following reduction of posterior derangement patients should be very careful when rising from the lying and sitting position to standing. Normally, the spine is momentarily flexed when standing up and this must now be prevented. Patients must be shown how to lordose when rising from lying and sitting, because without help they will not easily master this. Again, we must emphasise that even a momentary loss of lordosis may cause recurrence of the derangement.

If patients are uncomfortable while lying in bed, it may be advisable to sleep with a lumbar supportive roll around the waist. This helps to maintain the lordosis when lying supine, and prevents the spine from sagging when lying on the side. On awaking the next morning the patient may feel stiff and painful, but after about an hour he will loosen up and find himself much improved compared with the previous day.

The second treatment should be given twenty-four hours after the first session. Only after this time may we confirm that we have made the correct diagnosis and have chosen the correct principle of treatment. *If on returning the patient reports improvement,* there is usually a definite change in the symptoms — that is, the pain has centralised or decreased in intensity; or its frequency is reduced; or both. Examination of the range of extension reveals improvement and the patient is better indeed. Our diagnosis is confirmed and we should continue with extension principle procedures. It is a basic rule of treatment, applicable to all syndromes, that *technique presently resulting in improvement should not be added to, modified or replaced in any way until all improvement ceases.* Thus, the same procedures can be continued safely over a number of days, provided the symptoms continue to improve. When the patient no longer has constant pain he may discontinue lying prone and lying prone in extension (**Proc. 8:1 and 8:2**). His intermittent pain is now most likely caused by loss of the lordosis, especially in slouched sitting, and we must emphasise the importance of the correct sitting posture once more. At this stage the introduction of the slouch overcorrect procedure is desirable in order that the patient may fully appreciate that slouched sitting will produce low back pain whereas correct sitting abolishes it. As further improvement becomes apparent, extension in lying (**Proc. 8:3**) may be reduced to two or three times per day — preferably morning, noon and evening, and may be replaced during the day by extension in standing (**Proc. 8:6**) whenever it is felt necessary.

We must warn the patient that after having started the treatment programme he is likely to experience 'new pains'. These may be felt higher in the back, between the shoulder blades, and possibly in the arms. They are different from the original pain for which treatment was sought, and are the result of adjustment by the body to new positions and movements. New pains should be expected and will wear off in a few days to a week, provided the exercises are continued.

All patients should be instructed that, if they have severe pain which worsens or peripheralises at the time of exercising, they should stop the exercises and ask further advice. We must make sure it is well understood that, to be guilty of aggravation of symptoms, the exercises must actually increase the pain *at the time of performance* and not two hours afterwards. Pain felt immediately after exercising can be a result of the exercise. Pain appearing two hours afterwards is commonly felt because of the position occupied at that time — for example, sitting slouched while watching television.

I have outlined this far the routine that should apply in most Derangement One patients and which should result in the rapid and uneventful resolution of the symptoms. However symptoms and signs do not always respond as we would wish. Where reduction of posterior derangement proves difficult it becomes necessary to apply progressively increasing stresses in order to achieve reduction, and there is a certain order in which these progressions should be made.

Let us assume that the patient already described as an example does not continue to improve, that after the first twenty-four hours improvement ceases. Either the self applied reduction stresses are not adequate to fully reduce the derangement or our diagnosis may be incorrect or the patient may have inadvertently or unwittingly caused recurrence of the derangement. Re-examination is necessary to exclude incorrect diagnosis and re-instruction necessary to ensure the patient understands the self treatment procedures especially those regarding posture, and reduction. Having excluded other possible causes for non-improvement we must conclude that therapist technique should be applied before self treatment procedures will again become effective.

Under normal circumstances repeated extension will result in a progressive reduction of pain and or centralisation will occur, but in this instance such a result is not forthcoming. Pain is not continuing to reduce and is still present at the maximum point of extension in lying (**Proc. 8:3**). *Whenever difficulty arises in obtaining reduction of Derangement One the following progressions should be applied.*

The first progression should be the application of extension mobilisation combined at intervals with rotation mobilisation in extension (**Proc. 8:7 and 8:9**) so that eight to ten of each is applied in succession to each segment indicated. As well as the affected segment, the segment above and below should be mobilised. This should immediately be followed by extension in lying (**Proc. 8:3**) which now will be increasing in range with concommitant reduction of or centralisation of pain. The effects of mobilisation will be apparent following twenty-four hours and if improvement has resulted the progression should be repeated.

The second progression should be applied only if the first progression has failed to reduce derangement. Again apply the technique of extension mobilisation (**Proc. 8:7**). After ten pressures to each of the appropriate segments maintain a continuous pressure at the level affected and ask the patient to perform about ten extension in lying movements (**Proc. 8:3**) against the pressure of your hands. Ensure your pressure is moderate but sufficient to prevent the pelvis moving from the treatment table. This increased stress surprisingly, (in derangement) permits freer painless movement rather than more difficult painful movement. This progression will frequently but not always remove the last obstruction to full extension. It may be necessary to apply these sequences on two or three successive days. Should reduction still be elusive a further progression may be required.

The third progression is the extension thrust manipulation (**Proc. 8:8**) and should only be applied if the preceding progressions have failed. Prior to manipulation, extension mobilisation (**Proc. 8:7**) and rotation mobilisation in extension (**Proc. 8:9**) should be applied in order to relax the patient and to provide the therapist with the necessary pre-manipulative information. Remember that repeating the mobilisation should be centralising or reducing pain as the derangement reduces. Providing this is occuring the manipulation can be administered. Should peripheralisation or increasing pain appear then the manipulation is inappropriate. This information can only be acquired by pre-testing. If the manipulation is successful it is usually evident immediately, and further treatment at this session is inadvisable. The patient should proceed with the self treatment programme as instructed on the first visit.

Following each progression the patient should continue through the following twenty-four hours with all advice and exercises initially prescribed. It should be emphasised again here that the progressions should only be initiated when all improvement utilising the patients own movements and abilities have been exhausted. Do not touch the patient unless you are certain that reduction cannot be achieved by any other means.

It can safely be assumed that reduction of Derangement One has been accomplished when full maximum extension in lying is painless even though the patient may describe and be aware of a 'strain pain' in this position. It is my experience that patients are well able to differentiate the 'strain pain' from the pain that caused consultation. It is necessary *always* to ask them to make the differentiation, for when asked, 'in maximum extension do you have pain?', the answer in invariably 'yes' indicating to the unwary that the derangement is not reduced. However if you further ask 'is it pain, or strain' the answer is usually 'strain'. A very subjective line of questioning I know, but very important for I have seen therapists abandon the extension principle of treatment merely because the patient described a pain at the extreme of extension, that occurs commonly as end range strain in any normal joint.

Reduction of the derangement can be assumed when extension is painless. The patient may still describe a pain that appears when he sits and also a pain that appears when he flexes the lumbar spine past a certain point. This description can also be misleading and creates the impression that the derangement is still present. Posterior derangement cannot exist when extension is full and free and painless. The pain the patient is now describing appears in sitting and in flexion because the collagen laid down in the healing structures is now under stress as the posterior vertebral margins are separated by the action of slouching or flexing. These are not the pains of derangement, although derangement could perhaps develop if the positions are maintained for too long. These pains are the pains that arise from dysfunction and are now the sole cause of the remaining symptoms. If left untreated they can remain for years and cause end range pain whenever the patient moves to the extreme of flexion.

It appears that the first collagen fibres appear at about the fifth day after tissue damage occurs and these are the first foundations of scar tissue. Without movement this collagen will be laid down in a haphazard and disorderly fashion and as this disorderly structured tissue contracts with time an inelastic scar forms within the elastic annulus.

It is important that we recognise the signs that indicate when it is appropriate to commence the procedures that when applied enhance the quality of the developing collagen. By applying the appropriate stress, we can influence the direction in which the newly formed collagen fibres will lie so enhancing the strength and quality of the new tissue. At the same time we ensure that the scar that forms is an extensible scar and will not interfere with the adjacent still healthy annular structures. Function must always be restored following posterior derangement.

Recovery of full function

When commencing with flexion procedures initially only flexion in lying (**Proc. 8:13**) should be considered. Because of its additional gravitational stress flexion in standing (**Proc. 8:14**) should not be applied yet. To ensure that flexion in lying (**Proc. 8:13**) may be started safely reassessment of the test movement of flexion in lying is essential. The first time flexion in lying is performed it may cause pain as already some adaptive shortening has taken place in the posterior joint structures due to the maintenance of lordosis. *Flexion becoming more painful on repetition* indicates that it is too early to perform stretching in flexion; if continued, derangement is likely to recur or shortened structures may be damaged as a result of premature stretching. But *flexion becoming less painful on repetition* indicates that adaptively shortened structures are gradually being lengthened without further damage; flexion procedures may now be started.

In order to recover flexion the patient must commence with flexion in lying (**Proc. 8:13**). Because of the risks involved when performing flexion exercises following recent derangement, he should initially be careful and the following precautions must be taken:

When starting flexion in lying (**Proc. 8:13**) the patient should reduce the number of exercises performed at each session, as well as the frequency of the sessions per day — for example, five or six repetitions of the exercise should be done five or six times per day. Once the condition proves stable, he may gradually work towards a full programme of ten repetitions performed each hour or hour and a half.

Flexion in lying (**Proc. 8:13**) *must always be followed by extension in lying* (**Proc. 8:3**) to ensure that after exercising, the fluid nucleus is restored to the optimal position within the disc, thus removing the risk of recurrence. If due to circumstances the performance of extension in lying (**Proc. 8:3**) is impossible, extension in standing (**Proc. 8:6**) must be performed instead.

Flexion in lying (**Proc. 8:13**) should not be done during the first few hours of the day. In this time period the risk of incurring derangement is increased due to an increase in the volume of nuclear fluid as a result of reabsorption and imbibition properties of the disc. This has previously been discussed (Chapter 11).

When no further flexion can be gained with flexion in lying (**Proc. 8:13**) the patient should progress to flexion in standing (**Proc. 8:14**). The same precautions must be taken as for flexion in lying (**Proc. 8:13**). Thus, flexion in standing (**Proc. 8:14**) should be started on a reduced scale, should always be followed by extension in lying (**Proc. 8:3**) or extension in standing (**Proc. 8:6**) as a second choice, and should never be performed first thing in the morning. Once full flexion is recovered flexion in standing (**Proc. 8:14**) can be discontinued.

Recovery of flexion is considered to be complete when on performance of flexion in lying or standing full range of movement is achieved without pain, though a strain may be felt.

Prevention of Recurrence

Once recovery of function is achieved, the patient is advised to continue for at least six weeks, possibly longer, with extension in lying (**Proc. 8:3**) twice per day — early in the morning and late at night — flexion in lying (**Proc. 8:13**) once per day — late at night; extension in standing (**Proc. 8:6**) whenever necessary during the day; and the slouch-correct exercise whenever becoming negligent regarding the correct sitting posture.

Very few patients require to reduce or discontinue activities following derangement of the lumbar spine. We must explain to the patient that he may resume all the activities he is used to and enjoys doing — for example, sports activities, gardening, concreting, activities involving lifting — provided he follows the advice and instructions given to prevent recurrence of derangement. Prophylactic measures are outlined in detail in Chapter 14.

I believe that failure to prevent recurrence is often the result of *our failure* to restore full function following derangement or trauma; *our failure* to ensure the patient has adequate knowledge and full understanding of the prophylactic measures; and, not less often, the patient's failure to adhere to the prophylactic measures and to apply self-treatment procedures when these are called for.

TYPICAL TREATMENT PROGRESSION — DERANGEMENT ONE

Day one:
— Assessment and conclusion/diagnosis.
— Explanation of cause of derangement and treatment approach.
— Reduction of derangement: commence with lying prone, lying prone in extension, extension in lying.
— Instruct to maintain lordosis at all times, must sit with lordosis and insert lumbar support. May benefit from supportive roll in bed.
— Repeat extension procedures each hour to maintain reduction and prevent recurrence.
— If extension in lying is not possible, it must be replaced by extension in standing.
— On recurrence of symptoms watch maintenance of lordosis even more, and immediately perform extension in lying.
— Demonstrate the use of lumbar supports in sitting and lying.

Day two:
— Confirm diagnosis.
— Check sitting posture and exercises.
— If improving then change nothing other than reducing extension in lying to once every two hours; replace extension in lying with extension in standing when necessary.
— If no improvement at all then check vhat exercises are performed far enough into extension, often enough during the day, and that the lordosis is well kept.
— Add extension mobilisation, possibly rotation mobilisation in extension.
— Warn for 'new pains'.

Day three:
— Check sitting posture and exercises.
— If improving, continue with procedures as directed.
— Once constant pain has changed to intermittent pain, stop lying prone and lying prone in extension; start the slouch-over correct exercise.
— If no improvement, concentrate on mobilisation techniques and add extension manipulation.

Day four:

— Check exercises and progress.
— If progress is satisfactory, reduce treatment to three times per week.
— Continue with same programme until painfree for three days at least.
— If progress is unsatisfactory, repeat mobilisation and manipulation techniques.

Day five and seven:

— Check exercises and progress.
— Once painfree for three days reduce extension in lying to three times per day and replace it by extension in standing whenever necessary during the day.
— Commencing flexion in lying; take all necessary precautions.
— Flexion in lying *must* be followed by extension in lying.

Further treatments:

— I prefer to see patients with derangement every day until the reduction is stable and patients are in control. This may take up to five days. Then the treatment may be reduced to alternate days.
— Once reduction of derangement proves stable and the patient has been painfree for at least three days, flexion exercises may be started to recover function.
— All flexion exercises must be followed by extension in lying; if this is not possible extension in standing must be performed.
— When no further flexion can be gained with flexion in lying, the patient must start flexion in standing.
— When function is recovered flexion in standing may cease.
— The patient is advised to continue with the exercises for another six weeks to prevent recurrence: he will do extension in lying in the morning; flexion in lying followed by extension in lying in the evening; extension in standing whenever necessary during the day; and possibly the slouch-overcorrect exercise, whenever becoming negligent regarding sitting.
— Before discharge prophylaxis and self-treatment must be discussed in detail. We must emphasise that *self-treatment is infinitely preferable to dependence on therapy.*

DERANGEMENT TWO:

Central or symmetrical pain across L4/5.
With or without buttock and/or thigh pain.
With deformity of lumbar kyphosis (Fig. 12:1).

This acute disturbance within the disc is a progression of Derangement One and, if handled incorrectly, can easily be converted into an acute lateral shift with predominence of unilateral pain (Derangement Four). Any applied torsion will cause this derangement to increase laterally and must therefore be avoided.

Derangement Two gives us the clearest clinical picture, reflecting the phenomena occurring within the disc during derangement. There is excessive posterior accumulation of the nucleus with a major blockage of extension accompanying the deformity of acute lumbar kyphosis. Not only is extension prohibited, the vertebrae are also forced apart and their posterior margins cannot approximate. Any attempt to do so results in severe pain, the patient being forced to return to the flexed position where he finds some temporary relief.

Fig. 12:1.
Treatment of Derangement Two from start to finish.

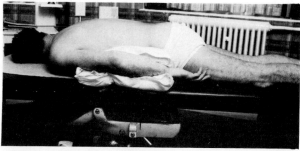

Commence reduction by allowing the patient to lie in slight flexion. Two pillows support the spine.

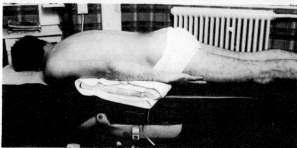

Now one pillow supports lumbar flexion.

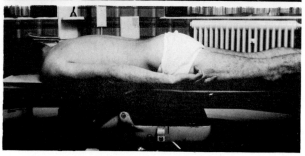

With no support the lordosis is beginning to appear.

Fig. 12:1 (continued)

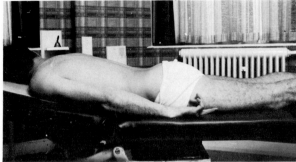

*The spine moves towards
more extension.*

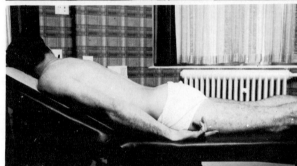

As the couch is raised . . .

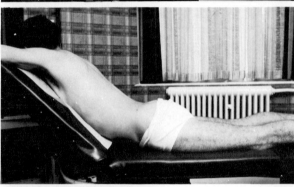

*. . . extension increases until
the . . .*

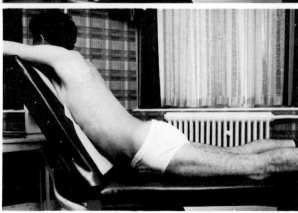

. . . lordosis is fully restored.

Fig. 12:1. (continued)

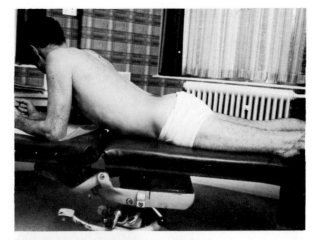

After resting flat for a minute or two, the patient should . . .

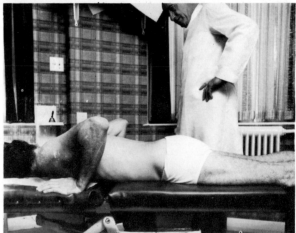

. . .then apply the extension . . .

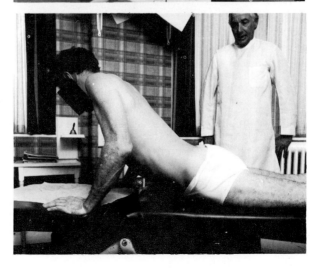

. . . movements himself . . .

Fig. 12:1. (continued)

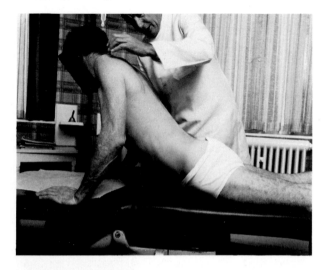

... and remember that the
lumbar ...

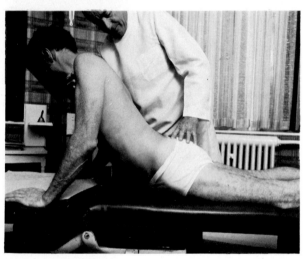

... spine must sag into full
relaxation in order to obtain
the maximum effect.

Treatment

The management of the patient with Derangement Two must be meticulous in
the first treatment session. Due to the blockage of extension the patient is
normally unable to lie prone, and this is a major obstacle to reduction. The self-
treatment procedures of the derangement syndrome can only be commenced
when the patient can comfortably lie prone.

In order to effectively treat the kyphotic derangement we must gradually
reduce the kyphosis until the prone position is attained. Only then will the
patient be able to start the procedures recommended in the treatment of
Derangement One. Place the patient prone, ensuring the lumbar spine remains
in flexion by placing pillows under the abdomen. The pillows are then gradually
withdrawn, one at a time at five minute intervals or as tolerated, until the patient

reaches the prone position. To facilitate a slow and gradual reduction it is wise to use several small pillows rather than one or two big ones. An adjustable treatment couch is extremely valuable and much preferred to the use of pillows.

Time, the important factor so often overlooked, is essential in the reduction of Derangement Two. To reduce the deformity of kyphosis up to 45 minutes must be allowed for the fluid nucleus to alter its silhouette and its position within the disc. If reduction pressures are applied gradually, allowing intervals between each progression towards extension, a slow but observable recovery of movement will occur. Too rapid increases in the extension range will cause severe pain and may provoke immediate regression.

Once the patient is able to lie horizontally without severe pain and providing the centralisation phenomenon is occuring an attempt should be made to develop the treatment along the lines recommended for Derangement One. Should the level of pain produced by extension in lying (**Proc. 8:3**) be still so severe as to prevent its use we must utilise sustained extension procedures. (**Proc. 8:5**) The progressions should be small and gradual, the patients shoulders being lifted perhaps four to five centimetres at a time.

On first raising the couch the patient will experience an increase in symptoms and providing these are consistent with the criteria applying to centralisation it is safe to proceed. After a few minutes in the higher position the pain should start to reduce in the thigh or buttock, and although it may increase centrally near the lumbar four five area this should not last for more than a minute or so. Once the pain has subsided to its former level, then and only then can progression to the next higher level be made. Should the centralised pain fail to subside, return the patient for a few minutes to the horizontal position and allow him to recover from the stresses, which can be rather trying. Once recovered, repeat the extension progressions (**Proc. 8:5**) which second time around are normally much easier to tolerate. Each progressive increase in extension will initiate the cycle of pain increase, followed by centralisation of pain, followed by a gradual reduction in the central or near central intensity.

It may be necessary from time to time during the course of the reduction to allow the patient a few minutes in the prone relaxed position to permit recovery from the stress of the sustained position. Following the recovery period it will now be possible to raise the patient rapidly to the former maximum extended position from which he has just rested. The impediment to obtaining extension is beginning to diminish.

Following the recovery of extension by this method (**Proc. 8:5**) we have reversed Derangement Two to One. The deformity and the pain referred to the buttocks and thigh should no longer be present. Treatment can proceed either immediately or on the following day as for Derangement One.

Pain and deformity of acute lumbar kyphosis can be significantly reduced in the first treatment session. If complete reduction is not possible, at least reduction to Derangement One is usually achieved. It is of vital importance to instruct the patient in the steps required to reduce the derangement himself in case of recurrence. If after returning home lying prone is too painful, the patient must repeat the sequence of lying over pillows and then gradually lowering himself until the prone position is obtained. This can be done on the floor over cushions or in bed over pillows. If reduction of derangement is maintained, the patient will usually be able to commence the extension principle procedures as for Derangement One the next day.

It may take up to twenty-four hours, occassionally longer, to reduce Derangement Two to Derangement One. Once this is accomplished treatment should progress on a daily basis *exactly as described for Derangement One,* and the recovery time will be the same as for patients with Derangement One.

DERANGEMENT THREE:

> Unilateral or asymmetrical pain across L4/5.
> With or without buttock and/or thigh pain.
> No deformity.

In Derangement Three the disturbance within the disc is located more postero-laterally rather than the postero-central position of Derangement One. This may be a progression of Derangement One, but it can also be the primary site of derangement.

Treatment

Initially the treatment should be the same as for Derangement One. The first twenty-four hours of treatment will determine whether the procedures for reduction of Derangement One can successfully be applied to Derangement Three. Very often the application of the extension principle for Derangement Three reduces the disturbance to Derangement One within twenty-four hours.

If on the second visit the patient is improving and the unilateral pain is reducing or centralising, or has moved evenly across the back, self-reduction is progressing and the extension principle as laid out for Derangement One must be continued.

On the second visit, should the patient show no improvement, re-examination and or re-instruction may be necessary; or, as was the case in the reduction of Derangement One the pressures may be inadequate. Should the applied reductive pressures prove inadequate it will again be necessary to progressively increase these and additionally alter the direction in which they may have to be applied.

The first progression in Derangement Three should be precisely the same as that applied as the first progression in the treatment of Derangement One. This progression should be given on the second day.

The second progression should be applied if the patient returns on the third day and is unimproved. With the patient in the prone position a lateral shift is formed by the therapist laterally gliding the patients pelvis away from the painful side. (This in effect creates a lateral shift towards the painful side.) With the pelvis in this off centre position the patient should be asked to perform a sequence of extension in lying (**Proc. 8:3**). There is often an initial centralisation of pain as the extensions are commenced. Should the pain subsequently move laterally or peripherally it may be necessary for the therapist to maintain the off centre position passively as the extensions are performed. Once the repetition of extension results in reduction of pain, or pain felt consistently in the mid line, the therapist can release the passive maintenance of the shifted pelvis. Providing the pains are now reduced or remaining centrally, treatment can progress as for the reduction of Derangement One. It is important to teach the patient how to place the pelvis laterally on his own, for he may have to make this lateral correction at home, in order for extension in lying to be effective.

(An early indication that this progression may be necessary is often obtained during the course of examination of the test movements. Where lateral gliding in standing increases or decreases the patients symptoms or where these movements cause the initiation of centralisation it can be assumed that progression two in Derangement Three is likely to succeed.)

The patient should apply the second progression during the performance of the self treatment procedure of extension in lying (**Proc. 8:3**) whenever he does these during the next twenty-four hours.

The third, fourth and fifth progressions should be applied if on the fourth day there is still no improvement.

The third progression sustained rotation, (**Proc. 8:11**) should be applied and its effects recorded. The patients legs should be moved towards the painful side as the first rotation is applied. (My records indicate that pressure applied in this direction is most consistently followed by rapid improvement. The centralisation phenomenon is the ultimate guide however.) The position should be held for up to two minutes depending on the patients tolerance and centralisation.

The fourth progression should be rotation manipulation in extension (**Proc. 8:10**).

The fifth progression should be rotation manipulation in flexion (**Proc. 8:12**).

Centralisation or reduction of pain must always be our guide regarding the side to which the technique should be performed or pressure applied. It is my experience that manipulation has a rapid effect and if there is no change in the symptoms after two manipulations in one direction, performed on successive days, the technique should be applied in the opposite direction provided centralisation and reduction of pain occur.

Once full centralisation is achieved Derangement Three is reversed to Derangement One. The treatment should now be continued and progressed exactly as for Derangement One.

DERANGEMENT FOUR:

> Unilateral or asymmetrical pain across L4/5.
> With or without buttock and/or thigh pain.
> With deformity of lumbar scoliosis (Fig. 12:2).

In 1956 I was fortunate enough to observe an acute lumbar scoliosis in a patient friend, who had more than the average faith in my ability as well as an intense fear of remaining deformed for life. The lateral shift with which he presented was more generous than usually seen, and the poor fellow was in great trouble indeed. At that time I did not know of any treatment method which would restore him rapidly to normal, and there did not appear to be any such reference in the literature either. My friend's desire to become painfree, his intense fear of remaining deformed for life coupled with my own curiosity regarding the mechanism causing the scoliosis led me to an abortive attempt to rectify the problem and correct the lateral shift. Needless to say, my friend was no better as a result but he was no worse either. He had to retire to his bed for ten days, and four weeks later he was painfree.

I tell this story for a specific reason. The fact that my friend left me neither better nor worse was of little concern to me at the time. However, the fact that his right sided pain had become left sided and the tilt of his trunk to the left had changed to the right, caused great consternation. I wondered what possible pathology could behave in this manner. In the only book available at that time to assist in the treatment of spinal disorders, Cyriax[24] provided the clue that the intervertebral disc is the most likely structure to be responsible for the lateral shift phenomenon.

From then on, bearing the disc in mind, I closely observed every lateral shift that presented and attempted to reduce the derangement. For two years I was unsuccessful, regularly bringing patients to the upright position only to hopelessly watch them fall back into scoliosis. It was not until the significance of facet apposition in extension occurred to me, that I applied the extension principle following lateral shift correction to ensure maintenance of the erect posture.

In the past ten years I have had ample opportunity to treat patients in many parts of the world. On such occasions I am always provided with lateral shift patients who failed to respond to other treatment methods. *Apart from the patients whose lateral shift had been present for too long,* most responded rapidly and well to my correction techniques. In general, no more than four days are required to reduce the deformity of scoliosis. The procedure of lateral shift correction has now been adopted by doctors and therapists in many parts of the world.

Derangement Four

Many theories have been put forward to explain the symptoms and peculiar behaviour of the derangement presented. These theories involve either disc, facet joint, ligaments and muscles, or combinations of any of these structures.

Because in its most extreme form the lateral shift co-exists with a prolapsed intervertebral disc exhibiting an accomplished protrusion, we can assume that the disc is heavily involved in the production of this deformity. It is my opinion that Derangement Four is a lateral progression of the posterior disc disturbance of Derangement Two, and a simple progression of Derangement Three.

There is evidence that the incidence of deformity of scoliosis is higher in men than in women. My own statistics show that of all the patients presenting with a lateral shift in a certain time period seventy percent were male and thirty percent female.[12] The results of a similar study reports a proportion of ninety percent male to only ten percent female patients.[41]

Although the literature reports an even distribution of back pain among the sexes, I would dispute this, in patients with the derangement syndrome.

Does the rather more accentuated lordosis of the female have anything to do with a lower incidence of lumbar scoliosis?

The majority of patients are seen to develop a lateral shift away from the painful side. My statistics show that ninety percent behave in this fashion, whereas the remaining ten percent deviate towards the painful side.[12] In the latter group reduction is much more difficult to achieve and recovery may take up to three times longer than in patients of the first group.

A small number of patients exhibit an alternating scoliosis. I believe that when a minor disc bulge exists close to the midline very little movement can under certain circumstances cause the bulging to move to the opposite side, again occupying a postero-lateral position. As the disc bulge changes position the lateral shift deformity resulting from the bulge will also change sides. The patient under examination can sometimes create the alternating deformity at will, once he has observed its nature and the mechanism effecting it.

The incidence of a relevant lateral shift in patients with low back pain is very high. My statistics show that fifty-two percent of patients with low back pain have a relevant lateral shift[10] that is, alteration of the lateral shift causes a change in intensity or site of pain or both.

The significance of derangement with deformity of scoliosis is much greater than is generally recognised. In the presence of a lateral shift either flexion or extension in the lumbar spine may be impaired, and sometimes both are affected. Lateral flexion to one side is similarly reduced. The loss of movement is always visible, sometimes markedly so. Furthermore, patients with even a minor lumbar scoliosis who are extended by exercises, mobilisation or manipulation, will become significantly worse with enhancement and peripheralisation of pain. The application of an extension thrust manipulation to a patient with a barely discernable lateral shift may precipitate a disc prolapse. Many patients with an undetected minor lateral shift have entered a clinic for treatment of their back pain only to walk out with sciatica. Again, I must emphasise that it is necessary to test all patients with low back pain for evidence of a relevant lateral shift.

I believe that, to a large extent, the disrepute surrounding the application of extension exercises has developed because of failure to detect minor lumbar scolioses and determine their relevance to symptoms. Indeed, many extension procedures are not successful due to lack of understanding of the nature of the condition to be treated. Usually extension fails because:

(1) not enough time is allowed for reversal of nuclear fluids to take place;
(2) it is done actively instead of passively;
(3) a lateral shift is present;
(4) or it is applied in the presence of extension dysfunction which results in the production of pain and the abandonment of the exercise.

Fig. 12:2. *Treatment of Derangement Four from start to finish.*

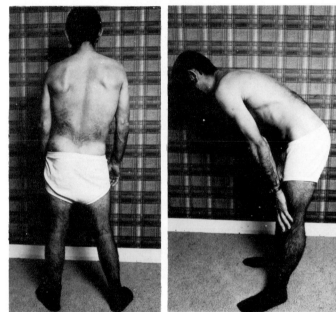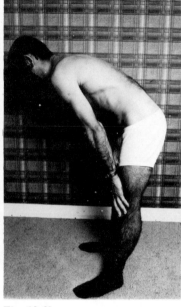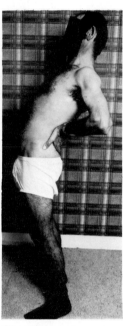

Fig. 12:2a.　　　　　　**Fig. 12:2b.**　　　　　　**Fig. 12:2c.**

Fig. 12:2d.

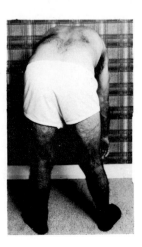

Fig. 12:2a. *Examination of standing posture — primary lateral shift.*

Fig. 12:2b. *Examination of movement — flexion in standing.*

Fig. 12:2c. *Examination of movement — extension in standing.*

Fig. 12:2d. *Examination of movement — deviation in flexion.*

Fig. 12:2. (continued)

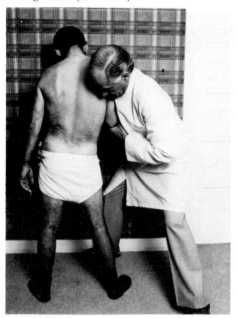

Fig. 12:2e.   **Fig. 12:2f.**

Correction of primary lateral shift.

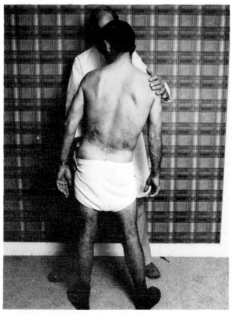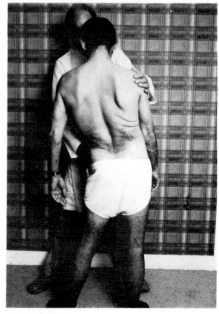

Fig. 12:2g.   **Fig. 12:2h.**

Teaching of self-correction of primary lateral shift.

Fig. 12:2 (continued)

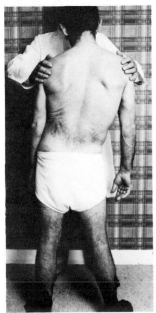 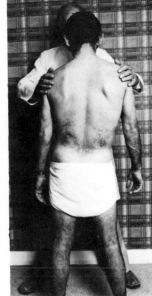 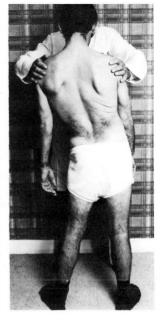

Fig. 12:2i.   **Fig. 12:2j.**   **Fig. 12:2k.**

Self-correction of primary lateral shift.

Recovery of extension.

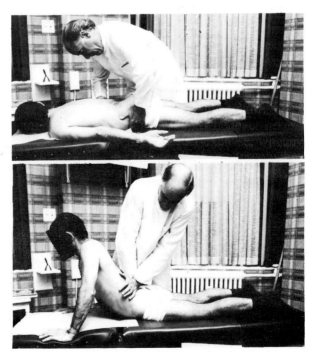

Fig. 12:2l.
*Overcorrection of primary
lateral shift — lying prone.*

Fig. 12:2m.
*Assisting maximum
extension.*

Fig. 12:2. (continued)

Recovery of extension
(continued)

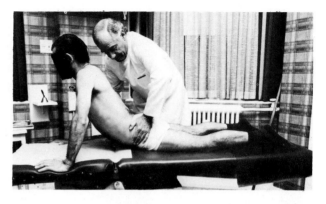

Fig. 12:2n.
*Overcorrection of primary
lateral shift in maximum
extension.*

Treatment

The acute lumbar scoliosis is a fascinating condition to treat. In general, the derangement is easily corrected when treated in the early stages, but becomes more difficult to reduce as time passes. After twelve weeks reduction becomes virtually impossible,[12] and if at this time marked deformity is still present it is usually permanent unless the affected disc is surgically removed. Even then a minor residual lateral shift often remains visible.

The techniques I developed in the late 1950's for the correction of lumbar scoliosis and first described in 1972,[12] are still the most effective in the treatment of patients with Derangement Four. Despite many efforts to improve the basic procedure this has not been altered in any significant way. I have made some minor changes in the method of achieving correction and these have been included in the discussion of the procedure (**Proc. 8:16**).

In a patient with Derangement Four the lateral shift must be corrected first (**Proc. 8:16**). Once correction or, if possible, slight overcorrection is achieved the extension loss must be restored (**Proc. 8:3**) and the lordosis maintained to prevent recurrence. Facet apposition makes lateral deviation impossible. Therefore, if the lordosis is maintained neither the lateral shift nor the pain will reappear.

It is of vital importance that the patient is shown on the very first visit how to maintain the lordosis and how to perform self-correction of his lateral shift (**Proc. 8:17**) in case of recurrence.

If the lateral shift has been corrected, but after a few days full centralisation is not yet achieved, the application of unilateral techniques may be indicated as outlined before (Derangement Three).

Once the lateral shift has been corrected and full centralisation is achieved as well Derangement Four is reversed to Derangement One. From now on the treatment must be continued and progressed exactly as described for Derangement One.

Effects of lateral shift correction on the disc

Farfan[26] has considered at length the possible effects on the vertebral structures that may result from spinal manipulation. He states that roto-scoliosis — or lateral shift — is caused by rotation usually occurring at the fourth and fifth lumbar vertebrae. He believes that the McKenzie technique of lateral shift correction is effective because firstly it opens the intervertebral space laterally in association with a slight flexion movement which is then followed by an extension movement in the lumbar spine. This produces reduction of the disc disturbance in a manner similar to squeezing a melon seed.

In my experience correction of many hundreds of lateral shifts has only on a few occasions caused a 'pop'-like effect. When perceivable the correction appears to be a slow flowing process rather than the effects one would associate with squeezing the melon seed. Whatever the true mechanics eventually prove to be, correction of lumbar scoliosis usually leads to a rapid reduction of deformity and symptoms with a corresponding restoration of function. Straight-leg-raising, if reduced before correction, is frequently dramatically restored to normal. I believe that the side bending deformity occurring with lumbar scoliosis is responsible for the reduction in straight-leg-raising on the painful side when the lateral shift is away from the painful side. In this case the elongation caused by the side bending deformity towards the painfree side will reduce the available root length range in straight-leg-raising. Thus, it is not necessarily a bulge in the annulus which limits straight-leg-raising. If the nucleus is disturbed enough to lead to the deformity of lumbar scoliosis without causing the outer annulus to bulge, the deformity by itself will be responsible for the nerve root tension.

Farfan[26] has stated that the procedure of straight-leg-raising does not necessarily have to stretch the sciatic nerve. There is enough evidence to suggest that reduced straight-leg-raising can be caused by a tight nerve root due to the rotation deformity as in sciatic or, as he prefers to call it, roto-scoliosis. This would partially explain why straight-leg-raising can quickly and simply be increased and reduced merely by laterally altering the patient's position in supine prior to performing the test. Under these circumstances the objectivity of straight-leg-raising is suspect, and the test is therefore irrelevant in judging progress.

It should be pointed out that testing of straight-leg-raising can be very misleading and is only reliable as an objective guide when the patient has constant sciatic pain. Constant sciatic pain is caused by constant mechanical deformation. When a disc protrusion is of sufficient magnitude to cause constant compression of the nerve root, alteration of the lateral shift while lying supine will not allow a better range of straight-leg-raising. If there is constant sciatic pain and straight-leg-raising improves as a result of some manoeuvre, a reduction in the magnitude of the protrusion must have occurred following this manoeuvre. Under these circumstances the objectivity of straight-leg-raising remains constant and therefore the test is useful in assessing the value of a certain procedure and judging progress.

If there is intermittent sciatic pain, the pressure on the nerve root is intermittent. In this case a minor annular bulge may be influenced by movements and the patient's symptoms can be created or abolished at will without significant alteration in his condition.

DERANGEMENT FIVE:

> Unilateral or asymmetrical pain across L4/5.
> With or without buttock and/or thigh pain.
> With leg pain extending below the knee.
> No deformity.

Derangement Five is a straight progression of Derangement Three. In Derangement Five the magnitude and location of the disc disturbance are such that impingement of the nerve root and dural sleeve occurs, but is not sufficient to force deformity. If the history is of recent onset, the patient must be treated with great care. It is essential to determine whether the sciatica is constant or intermittent, because the treatment will be different accordingly. If the sciatica has been present for several weeks or months, as sometimes occurs, constant leg pain may have altered to intermittent pain. Generally, if the patient presents with a deformity of scoliosis, sciatica is likely to be constant, and if there is no deformity, sciatica is usually intermittent. Thus, Derangement Five patients are more likely to have intermittent sciatica though exceptions occur, expecially in acute stages of derangement.

Intermittent sciatica

Usually, the patient with Derangement Five presents without a deformity in the lumbar spine and the sciatica will be intermittent — that is, there are times in the day when the sciatica is not present. Neurological deficit is infrequently encountered in these patients as even short periods without root compression allow physiological recovery to some extent. Straight-leg-raising may or may not be limited.

If the root irritation is indeed intermittent, the patient can be treated with some caution using mechanical therapy. In the treatment we must make use of those positions and movements which are found to reduce or abolish the sciatica. It must be emphasised that any position or movement which produces or enhances sciatica should not be further developed. When neurological deficit is present the chances of success are greatly reduced.

Intermittent sciatica may be caused by a small disc bulge which is, depending on the patient's activities, alternately protruding into the canal and retreating into the disc substance,[13] but is not large enough to force deformity upon the joint.

Intermittent sciatica may also be caused by an adherent nerve root or entrapment which is placed under increased tension when certain movements are performed and positions are adopted. For example, a patient with sciatica may have recovered recently from an acute disc prolapse and his symptoms are now becoming intermittent; we must determine whether his sciatica is caused by an increase of disc bulging or by an increased nerve root tension due to entrapment, adherence or scarring; and when adherence of the nerve root is thought to be the cause, we must determine whether it is safe at this stage to stretch the nerve root without causing further disc prolapse.

To differentiate between sciatica caused by compression from a disc bulge, or that due to increased root tension from adherence, careful assessment of the flexion test movements is essential. Flexion in standing will enhance the sciatica in both situations — that is, in derangement and in root adherence. The answer to the problem will be found in flexion in lying, which will *not enhance sciatica in a patient with an adherent root, but will always enhance it when the disc is in a weakened state.* Thus, production or enhancement of sciatica which remains worse as a result of performing flexion in lying indicates that the increase in mechanical deformation is caused by a bulging disc. With such a response to the test movements it is dangerous for the patient to perform flexion exercises in standing as well as in lying, as this may lead to recurrence or increase of derangement.

Treatment

Should testing of flexion in lying indicate that sciatica is caused by a disc derangement and the disc wall is able to distend during this movement, it is likely that testing of extension in lying will have the opposite effect and reduce the derangement. If this is the case the patient must be placed under the extension principle for a period of twenty-four hours to confirm the diagnosis. If after this time there is a positive response to extension, the extension principle may be continued and the patient must be treated as for Derangement Three. If the response to extension appears to be negative, or if progress appears to be slow, the use of unilateral mobilisation and manipulation procedures is indicated as outlined before (Derangement Three). It will be understood that, once full centralisation is obtained treatment should be continued and progressed exactly as described for Derangement One.

Should the test movements indicate that sciatica is caused by entrapment — root adherence or scarring, the treatment described for this under Derangement Six should be applied. Remember however that the treatment must be considered to be that required for dysfunction. The derangement stage has now passed and the damage repaired.

DERANGEMENT SIX:

> Unilateral or asymmetrical pain across L4/5.
> With or without buttock and/or thigh pain.
> With leg pain extending below the knee.
> With deformity of sciatic scoliosis. (Fig. 12:3)

Derangement Six clearly is a progression of Derangement Four and Five. The patient commonly exhibits a sciatic scoliosis as well as a reduced lordosis. The sciatica is more likely to be constant and there is little chance of reducing the symptoms by positioning or movement. Often the patient states that movement brings relief of pain; however, movement or a change of position gives a short-lived respite only. Neurological deficit commonly occurs.

If in a patient with Derangement Six and constant sciatica most test movements are found to enhance the leg pain and no movement reduces it, a provisional diagnosis of accomplished disc protrusion can be made provided the presence of neurological deficit and a positive myelogram support this finding. Remember, that at this stage the condition is irreversible using mechanical therapy. Subsequent surgery usually confirms our diagnosis.

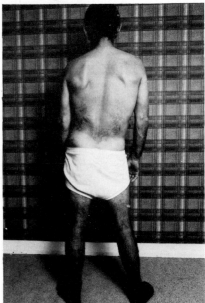

Fig. 12:3.
Patient with Derangement Six. This patient shows a similar deformity as the patient with Derangement Four — a primary lateral shift.

Constant sciatica

If there is no position in which the patient is painfree, we must be careful when sending the patient home on bed rest. It is certainly not desirable that the patient assumes positions which increase the symptoms. Before placing a patient on bed rest we must examine the various positions and their effects on sciatica and low back pain, and advise the patient accordingly. If there is a position which produces significant reduction in leg pain, the patient should be instructed to adopt and maintain that position for long periods at a time.

If no test movements or positions can be found to reduce the pain referred below the knee then, I believe, there are no techniques available which will have a beneficial effect on the derangement. Intermittent traction in the order of twenty minutes a day on an out-patient basis has been described as useful, but if progress is made it is difficult to attribute this to the treatment rather than to the passage of time. Continuous traction in bed is a different matter and often produces good enough results to make the procedure an attractive alternative to surgery.

Treatment

If test movements indicate that reduction of the derangement is possible, treatment should be commenced following the lines of that for Derangement Four and Five. During the treatment great care should be taken to check regularly if there is a change in peripheral symptoms. Increased tingling or numbness felt in the foot must never be ignored, and if these are present treatment should be modified immediately.

If there is improvement but full centralisation has not yet been achieved, the application of mobilising and manipulation procedures may be indicated. Techniques outlined previously (Derangement Three) may be utilised, provided *pre-manipulative testing is performed to ensure centralisation of symptoms is taking place.* If peripheral pain is enhanced in the pre-manipulative testing position, the manipulation should not be performed. Whatever procedure you have in mind, *never* manipulate a patient without pre-manipulative testing.

Should lateral shift correction produce reduction of the derangement, then progress usually is uncomplicated and treatment should continue as outlined for Derangement Four. The recovery of full flexion or the treatment of any residual flexion dysfunction must be delayed much longer after the resolution of a severe sciatica than is usually the case with pure lumbar pain. I consider eight to ten weeks from the time of onset of peripheral symptoms to be the minimum time before implementing the flexion dysfunction procedures to the maximum.

Stretching of adherent nerve root

Once the acute episode has subsided and the patient is able to attend to his occupation, nerve root adherence as a result of scarring may cause a persistent sciatic reference which, in some cases, may last for years. This disability will not produce neurological deficit if the initial episode has not already done so. It is desirable to reduce the nerve root entrapment or adherence, and in many patients this may be done successfully by using the procedures for flexion dysfunction — that is, the shortened structures should be stretched frequently and firmly every day until the adherence is resolved. To achieve this flexion in lying (**Proc. 8:13**) should be regularly performed for one week. This is followed by flexion in standing (**Proc. 8:14**) which must be performed often enough to elongate and stretch scarred and adherent tissue without causing further bulging of the disc wall (Fig. 12:4).

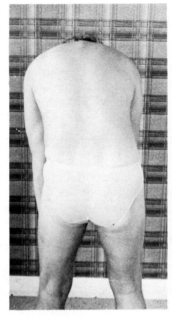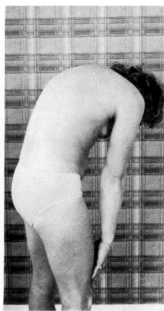

Fig. 12:4.
Treatment of adherent sciatic nerve root, using flexion in standing.

When treatment of dysfunction due to an adherent nerve root is commenced it should not be attempted during the first four to five hours of the day. During this time period the disc is likely to be under increased pressure as a result of its nocturnal imbibition and reabsorbtion of fluid. I recommend that in the initial stages of treatment the patient performs ten repetitions of flexion in standing (**Proc. 8:14**) from midday on, every three hours until retirement. When the derangement appears stable and the integrity of the disc wall is established, the patient may commence the exercise a little earlier in the day and repeat it every two hours. However, it is inadvisable to perform flexion in standing (**Proc. 8:14**) on awaking.

Because flexion in standing (**Proc. 8:14**) places stress on the disc wall and forces the disc posteriorly, there are always risks involved in stretching an adherent nerve root, especially in the initial stages. Therefore, flexion in standing (**Proc. 8:14**) must always and immediately be followed by extension in lying (**Proc. 8:3**), or if this is not possible by extension in standing (**Proc. 8:6**).

As the nerve root stretching becomes effective, the patient may perceive the same amount of pain whereas his flexion range has increased. Gradually his fingertips will move closer to his ankles, and where a certain amount of flexion produced significant pain before it may have become painfree now. It will become easier to drive the car and to walk uphill.

It is my belief that *intermittent* stress applied to joints in this manner strengthens ligamentous structures rather than damages them, while scar tissue will stretch and yield to such stress.[45] However, if a *sustained* stress is applied damage may occur to both ligamentous and scar tissue.

DERANGEMENT SEVEN:

Symmetrical or asymmetrical pain across L4/5.
With or without buttock and/or thigh pain.
With deformity of accentuated lumbar lordosis (Fig. 12:5).

In Derangement Seven the disturbance within the disc appears to be located in a more antero-lateral or anterior position, which leaves the patient with an accentuated lordosis as the presenting deformity. This type of derangement is not common, but it is easily identified.

The patient with Derangement Seven may exhibit such a gross loss of flexion that in full flexion the lumbar spine remains lordotic. At first sight the condition appears to be the common flexion dysfunction presenting with an accentuated lordosis. However, the patient describes a sudden onset of pain and assures that he was able to touch his toes easily the day before the onset of pain.

Fig. 12:5. *Patient with Derangement Seven.*

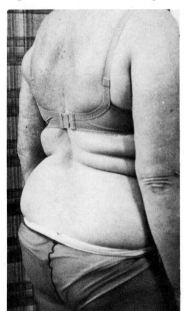

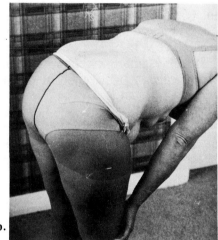

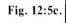
Fig. 12:5b.

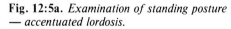
Fig. 12:5a.   Fig. 12:5c.

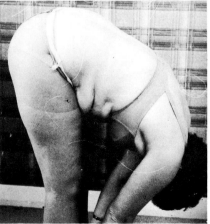

Fig. 12:5a. *Examination of standing posture — accentuated lordosis.*

Fig. 12:5b. *Flexion loss at commencement of treatment session.*

Fig. 12:5c. *Recovery of flexion at finish of* **same** *treatment session. The remarkable recovery of flexion within a short time period indicates derangement.*

Treatment

If examination shows a marked deviation in flexion, it may be necessary to perform flexion in step standing **(Proc. 8:15)** to reduce the lateral component of the derangement. Usually, this procedure rapidly brings the deviation to the midline. As soon as the deviation in flexion is corrected flexion in step standing **(Proc. 8:15)** should be discontinued. Correction of deviation in this type of derangement is sometimes very dramatic, and if the procedure is repeated too often the deviation in flexion may change to the opposite side. The treatment should be continued with flexion in lying **(Proc. 8:13)**.

If there is no deviation in flexion on the test movements, treatment should commence with flexion in lying **(Proc. 8.13)**, and after a few days flexion in standing **(Proc. 8:14)** may be added. Sometimes an intermediate stage of flexion seems indicated. This can be found by performing flexion in the sitting position and is progressed by placing the feet further from the chair as the flexion is performed. Once reduction of the derangement is achieved it is possible to recreate the derangement situation simply by performing extension in lying **(Proc. 8:3)**. This is exactly the opposite from the previous derangements with a posterior or postero-lateral disc disturbance where recurrence is to be expected as soon as the lordosis is lost following reduction.

If there is improvement but the patient has unilateral pain which has not fully centralised, the application of unilateral techniques may be indicated such as sustained rotation **(Proc. 8:11)** and rotation manipulation in flexion **(Proc. 8:12)**.

Because patients with deformity of accentuated lordosis rarely develop extension dysfunction, it is not necessary that extension procedures be included in the treatment of patients with Derangement Seven.

CHAPTER 13

Prophylaxis

The majority of patients responding to basic extension and flexion principles of treatment have been educated in the means of achieving pain relief and restoring function. They have carried out the self-treatment procedures and have to a large extent become independent of therapists. Following successful treatment it requires little emphasis to convince patients that if they were able to *reduce and abolish* pain already present, it should also be possible to *prevent the onset* of any significant future low back pain.

Of all the factors *predisposing* to low back pain only postural stresses can be easily influenced and fully controlled. We must develop this potential ingredient of prophylaxis to the full. The patient must understand that the risks of incurring low back pain are particularly great when the lumbar spine is held in sustained flexed positions; and that when the lordosis is reduced or eliminated for prolonged periods, *he must at regular intervals and before the onset of pain make a conscious effort to interrupt flexion, restore the lordosis and accentuate it momentarily to the maximum.* It is essential that the patient knows the reasons for doing this, and therefore we must explain to him in lay terms that on restoring the lordosis the intradiscal pressure decreases, the nuclear fluid moves anteriorly and the posterior stresses in and around the disc are reduced.

Briefly summarised, the following prophylactic measures should always be taken:

Prolonged sitting requires (a) maintenance of the lordosis by muscular control of the posture or, preferably, by insertion of a lumbar roll, (b) hourly interruption of sitting by standing up, walking around for a few minutes and accentuating the lordosis by a few repetitions of extension in standing (**Proc. 8:6**).

Activities involving prolonged stooping require (a) interruption of stooping at regular intervals by standing upright, (b) regularly reversing the curvature of the lumbar spine, restoring and accentuating the lordosis by a few repetitions of extension in standing (**Proc. 8:6**).

Lifting requires (a) the use of the correct lifting technique. Generally, if the object to be lifted exceeds fifteen kilograms, the strain must be taken with the lumbar spine in lordosis and the lift must be performed using the legs. If the object to be lifted weighs under fifteen kilograms less care is necessary, unless one has been in a bent or sitting position for some time prior to the lift. In the latter case the same rules apply as for lifting weights exceeding fifteen kilograms, (b) accentuation of the lordosis before and after lifting by a few repetitions of extension in standing **(Proc. 8:6)**.

If inadvertently pain has developed during sitting, stooping or lifting, the patient should immediately commence extension in lying **(Proc. 8:3)**. Extension in standing **(Proc. 8:6)**, very effective in preventing the onset of pain, is less effective when used to reduce present pain. *Extension in lying* **(Proc. 8 3)** *is the technique of first aid for back pain.*

Recurrence: At the first sign of recurrence the patient should immediately commence the procedures which previously led to recovery. Although an episode of low back pain can commence suddenly and without warning, many patients are aware of a minor degree of discomfort before the onset of severe pain. If this type of warning is given, the patient has an excellent chance to prevent the development of symptoms, provided the appropriate procedure is applied immediately.

It is not possible for patients to remember all verbal instructions and advice given during the first treatment. To avoid tedious repetition and to ensure the necessary information is conveyed to the patient, a list of instructions is supplied on the first visit. This list firstly deals with information for patients in the acute stage of low back pain, and secondly provides information required once recovery has taken place. These instructions form an important part of self-treatment, because when followed properly they will help in reduction of present symptoms and prevention of their recurrence.

WELLINGTON PHYSIOTHERAPY CLINIC

General Instructions — When in Acute Low Back Pain

You must retain the lordosis at all times (lordosis is the hollow in the lower back). Bending forwards as in touching the toes will only stretch and weaken the supporting structures of the back and lead to further injury. Losing the lordosis when sitting will also cause further strain.

SITTING
- When in acute pain you should sit as little as possible, and then only for short periods only.
- At all times you must sit with a lordosis. Therefore you must place a supportive roll in the small of the back, especially when sitting in a car or lounge chair.

- If you have the choice you must sit on a firm, high chair with a straight back such as a kitchen chair. You should avoid sitting on a low, soft couch with a deep seat; this will force you to sit with hips lower than knees, and you will round the back and lose the lordosis.
- The legs must never be kept straight out in front as in sitting in bed, in the bath or on the floor; in this position you are forced to lose the lordosis.
- When rising from sitting you must retain the lordosis; move to the front of the seat, stand up by straightening the legs, and avoid bending forwards at the waist.
- Poor sitting postures are certain to keep you in pain or make you worse.

DRIVING A CAR
- When in acute pain you should drive the car as little as possible. It is better to be a passenger than to drive yourself.

- When driving, your seat must be close enough to the steering wheel to allow you to maintain the lordosis. If in this position your hips are lower than your knees you may be able to raise yourself by sitting on a pillow.

BENDING FORWARDS
- When in acute pain you should avoid activities which require bending forwards or stooping, as you will be forced to lose the lordosis.
- You may be able to retain the lordosis by kneeling — for example, when making the bed, vacuuming, cleaning the floor, or weeding the garden.

LIFTING
- When in acute pain you should avoid lifting altogether.
- If this is not possible you should at least not lift objects that are awkward or heavier than about thirty pounds.
- You must always use the correct lifting technique: during lifting the back must remain upright and never stoop or bend forwards; stand close to the load, have a firm footing and wide stance; bend the knees and keep the back straight; have a secure grip on the load; lift by straightening the knees; take a steady lift and do not jerk; shift your feet to turn and do not twist your back.

LYING
- A good firm support is usually desirable when lying. If your bed is sagging, slats or plywood supports between mattress and base will firm it. You can also place the mattress on the floor, a simple but temporary solution.
- You may be more comfortable at night when you use a supportive roll. A rolled up towel, wound around your waist and tied down in front, is usually satisfactory.
- When rising from lying you must retain the lordosis; turn on one side, draw both knees up and drop the feet over the edge of the bed; sit up by pushing yourself up with the hands and avoid bending forwards at the waist.

COUGHING AND SNEEZING
- When in acute pain you must try to stand up, bend backwards and increase the lordosis while you cough and sneeze.

REMEMBER:
- At all times you must retain the lordosis; if you slouch you will have discomfort and pain.
- Good posture is the key to spinal comfort.

General Instructions — When Recovered From Acute Low Back Pain

You have recovered from the acute episode because of your ability to master the exercises which relieved your pain. These exercises must be repeated whenever situations arise which have previously caused pain. You must perform the corrective movements before the onset of pain. This is essential.

If you carry out the following instruction, you can resume your normal activities without the fear of recurrence.

SITTING
- When sitting for prolonged periods the maintenance of the lordosis is essential. It does not matter if you maintain this with your own muscles or with the help of a supportive roll, placed in the small of your back.

- In addition to sitting correctly with a lumbar support, you should interrupt prolonged sitting at regular intervals. On extended car journeys you should get out of the car every hour or two, stand upright, bend backwards five or six times, and walk around for a few minutes.

BENDING FORWARDS
- When engaged in activities which require prolonged forward bending or stooping — for example, gardening, vacuuming, concreting — you must stand upright, restore the lordosis and bend backwards five or six times before pain commences.
- Frequent interruption of prolonged bending by reversing the curve in the low back should enable you to continue with most activities you enjoy, even with some you do not enjoy.

LIFTING
- If the load to be lifted weighs over thirty pounds, the strain must be taken with the low back in lordosis and you must lift by straightening your legs.
- If the object weighs under thirty pounds less care is required, unless you have been in a bent or sitting position for some time prior to lifting. In the latter case you must lift as if the weight exceeds thirty pounds.
- In addition to correct lifting technique, you must stand upright and bend backwards five or six times after lifting.

RECURRENCE
- At the first signs of recurrence of low back pain you should immediately start the exercises which previously led to recovery, and follow the instructions given for when in acute pain.
- If this episode of low back pain seems to be different than on previous occasions, and if your pain persists despite following the instructions, you should contact a manipulative therapist.

REMEMBER:
- If you lose the lordosis for any length of time, you are risking recurrence of low back pain.

Robin McKenzie
16 The Terrace
Wellington

It seems that at this stage in the development of spinal therapy the responsibility for successful management and prophylaxis in low back pain lies with the manipulative therapist. As education is the only way of preventing low back pain induced and increased by poor posture, I would hope that in the future, prophylactic postural advice be provided at school level. This should really be the province of the physical education instructor, but unfortunately at the present time this profession does not yet have the necessary knowledge regarding prophylaxis for any spinal pain.

CHAPTER 14

Contra-Indications

Although it has been accepted throughout that all patients have received adequate medical screening, occasionally patients with serious pathology or mechanical disorders unsuited to mechanical treatment are encountered during routine examination. *If in the examination no position or movement can be found which reduces the presenting pain,* the patient is unsuited for mechanical therapy, at least at this time.

The existence of serious pathology should be considered when the history states that there has been no apparent reason for the onset of symptoms; that the symptoms have been present for many weeks or months, and have during that time increased in intensity; and that they are constant; and the patient feels that he is gradually getting worse. On examination the pain remains exactly the same, irrespective of positions assumed or movements performed. Usually there is little loss of function if any, and postural deformity is not often seen. In addition to the examination finding, the patient often looks unwell and may complain of feeling unwell. Mechanical procedures described in this book should never be applied to patients presenting with signs and symptoms of this nature.

Saddle anaesthesia and bladder weakness are indications of compression of the fourth sacral nerve root. These symptoms occur in major disc herniation and, when present, form a definite contra-indication to manipulative procedures.

Patients who exhibit signs of extreme pain — that is, who become transfixed on movement, and freeze and immobilise the spine when palpation is attempted — are considered unsuitable for mechanical therapy, at least at this stage.

Developmental or acquired anomalies of bone structures which may lead to weakness or instability of mechanical articulations are hazards to manipulative procedures. Architectural faults should be excluded from mechanical therapy. Exceptions are minor grades of spondylolisthesis where symptoms are mild and intermittent. The presence of spondylolisthesis at a certain segment is not necessarily an indication that symptoms are forthcoming from that segment. It is seen very often indeed that pain is the result of disc derangement at a different level.

A simple clinical test may determine whether spondylolisthesis is responsible for the presenting pain, as it will often reduce or abolish pain in the presence of that condition. Place one hand across the sacrum of the standing patient and the other firmly against the abdomen. By further compressing the abdominal content while at the same time increasing pressure on the sacrum, pain in standing arising from spondylolisthesis is markedly reduced or abolished. On the other hand, pain arising from derangement of any of the lumbar discs will usually be enhanced by this procedure, and postural or dysfunctional pain remains unaffected. Thus, if pain is increased with this test the patient should be treated as for the derangement syndrome, but if pain is reduced the presence of spondylolisthesis must be investigated and the necessary precautions must be taken in the treatment.

Bed rest

Patients with mechanical low back pain are often advised to rest as much as possible, preferably in bed. In many instances this is inappropriate if not bad advice. The nutrition of the intervertebral discs depends entirely on osmosis, and movements of the spine are essential for the flow of fluids containing nutriments. To rest the joints of patients with mechanical low back pain often only adds to the problems of restoration of function and full rehabilitation. The only patient who should be placed on bed rest is the *very acute patient with severe constant low back pain with or without sciatica whose symptoms are considerably worse during weight bearing, and in whom no movement or position can be found to reduce or centralise the pain.*

In order to prevent the development of dysfunction within or about the involved intervertebral joint following derangement, regular assessment of the patient on bed rest is required and treatment must be instituted as early as possible. This is particularly important in the patient who responds very well to bed rest, because without movement this patient will become painfree but may develop a significant loss of function.

Supports

If, following reduction of derangement, all efforts at prevention of immediate recurrence are unsuccessful, it may be desirable to supply the patient with a corset for *short term support and stability.* Long term use of a corset is undesirable as it merely hastens the development of dysfunction.

Surgery

The question of surgical intervention inevitably arises in the minds of doctors, therapists and patients alike when progress is slow or non-existent. The decision as to whether one should or should not operate must always concern the orthopaedic surgeon.

It is my experience that, in New Zealand, surgery will be performed only when conservative treatment methods have failed. This does not always include adequate mechanical therapy, but usually it has allowed adequate passage of time. Fortunately, few patients in New Zealand receive surgery for low back pain only, and the procedures of laminectomy and discectomy are reserved for patients suffering significant nerve root compression.

The difficulties surrounding the diagnostic criteria for surgical intervention are enormous. One study showed a large number of positive myelograms in lumbar spines of patients who were asymptomatic and had been admitted and X-Rayed for conditions other than low back pain.[5] Thus the value of the myelogram, the good old standby relied upon by many doctors, has become somewhat suspect.

The results of surgery can also be seen to vary significantly.[5] Randomly selected patients with low back pain, referred pain to one leg, and positive myelograms coupled with clinical signs, were divided into two groups. The patients in the one group received surgery, those in the other group not. It was found that at the end of one year ninety percent of the non-operated patients were better; that the operated patients were only better in the first two months following surgery; and that at the end of one year the results in the group that had received surgery were the same as in the group that had not been operated upon.

The final result of a disc lesion is not endangered by a three months' waiting period before surgery is undertaken. However, a longer wait may be prejudicial as it may leave the patient with residual disability.[5]

Fielding[5] states that Nachemson, Rothman and Hirsch have all found that there is a clear correlation between the early return of symptoms following surgery and the formation of scar tissue. Quoting Fielding:[5]

"Early return of symptoms usually means the formation of scarring which cannot be cured by surgery and means that the results will be poor".

Rothman[39] examined sixty-eight patients who had undergone two or more unsuccessful spinal surgical interventions. He reports that seventy-five percent of the patients claimed partial or total disability. Half of the failures in multiple surgery are due to scarring or nerve root adherence. Scarring and fibrosis are associated with a high failure rate and dismal results.

It is appropriate to make clear that scarring causes dysfunction, described earlier in this book. Scarring does not necessarily have to cause problems provided it is discovered early enough and dealt with adequately in the manner suggested in previous chapters. I believe that one procedure is mandatory following surgery for lumbar disc protrusion: that is, the regular performance of one full straight-leg-raising movement at two hourly intervals. This should reduce significantly the complications of fibrosis and nerve root adherence. Just as recent scars can be stretched and lengthened by dysfunction treatment procedures, so should the prevention of inextensible scar formation be feasible by the even earlier use of the same procedures.

References

[1] Fisk, J. W. (1977). "The painful neck and back". (Charles C. Thomas, Springfield, USA)

[2] Wood, P. H. N. (1976), "Epidemiology of back pain". in: "The Lumbar spine and back pain" ed. M. Jayson. (Pitman Medical Publishing Co., Turnbridge Wells, Great Britain)

[3] Anderson, J. A. D. (1976), "Back pain in industry". in: "The lumbar spine and back pain" ed. M. Jayson.

[4] Wyke, B. (1976), "Neurological aspects of low back pain". in: "The lumbar spine and back pain" ed. M. Jayson.

[5] Fielding, J. W. (1979), Orthopaedic and Physical Therapy Seminar, University of Cincinatti Medical Center, Sept. 1979.

[6.] La Rocca, H. and MacNab, I. (1969), "Value of pre-employment radiographic assessment of the lumbar spine", Canad. Med. Assoc. J. 101; 383.

[7] Nachemson, A. (1976), "A critical look at conservative treatment for low back pain". in: "The lumbar spine and back pain" ed. M. Jayson.

[8] Dixon, A.St.J. (1976), "Diagnosis of low back pain". in: "The lumbar spine and back pain" ed. M. Jayson.

[9] Magora, A. (1972), "Investigation of relation between low back pain and occupation", Ind. Med. Surg. 41; 5.

[10] McKenzie, R. A. (1979), "Prophylaxis in recurrent low back pain", NZ. Med. J. 89; 22.

[11] Andersson, B. J. G., et al. (1975), "The sitting posture: An electromyographic and discometric study", Orth. Cl. N. Am. Vol. 6, No. 1.

[12] McKenzie, R. A. (1972), "Manual correction of sciatic scoliosis", NZ Med. J. 76; 484.

[13] Shah, J. S., Hampson, W. G. H., and Jayson, M. I. V. (1978), "The distribution of surface strain in the cadaveric lumbar spine", J. Bone & Jt. Surg. 60B; 246.

[14] Armstrong, J. R. (1958), "Lumbar disc lesions" (E. & F. Livingstone Ltd., Edinburgh, London.)

[15] Andersson G. B. J., Murphy R. W., Ortengren R., and Nachemson A. (1979), "The influence of backrest inclination and lumbar support on lumbar lordosis", Spine, Vol. 4, No. 1; 52.

[16] Nachemson A. (1975), "Towards a better understanding of low back pain. A review of the mechanics of the lumbar disc", Rheum. & Rehab. 14; 129.

[17] Markolf K. L., and Morris J. M. (1974), "The structural components of the intervertebral disc. A study of their contributions to the ability of the disc to withstand compressive forces", J. Bone & Jnt. Surg. 56A; 675.

[18] Naylor A., and Shentall R. (1976), "Biochemical aspects of intervertebral discs in ageing and disease". in: "The lumbar spine and back pain" ed. M. Jayson.

[19] Nachemson A. (1976), "Lumbar intradiscal pressure". in: "The lumbar spine and back pain" ed. M. Jayson.

[20] Happey F. (1976), "A biophysical study of the human intervertebral disc" in: "The lumbar spine and back pain" ed. M. Jayson.

[21] Farfan H. F. (1973), "Mechanical disorders of the low back". (Lea & Febiger, Philadelphia, USA.)

[22] Fahrni W. H. (1976), , "Backache: Assessment and treatment". (Musqueam Publishers Ltd., Vancouver, Canada.)

[23] Vernon-Roberts B. (1976), "Pathology of degenerative spondylosis" in: "The lumbar spine and back pain" ed. M. Jayson.

[24] Cyriax J. (1969), "Textbook of orthopaedic medicine" Vol. 1, 5th ed. (Bailliere Tindall, London.)

[25] Charnley J. (1951), "Orthopaedic signs in the diagnosis of disc protrusion", Lancet cclx; 186.

[26] Farfan H. F. (1979), Orthopaedic and Physical Therapy Seminar, University of Cincinatti Medical Center, Sept. 1979.

[27] Park, W. M. (1976), "Radiological investigation of the intervertebral disc" in: "The lumbar spine and back pain" ed. M. Jayson.

[28] Yates A. (1976), "Treatment of back pain" in: "The lumbar spine and back pain" ed. M. Jayson.

[29] Jayson, M. I. V. (1976), Editor's Preface in: "The lumbar spine and back pain" ed. M. Jayson.

[30] Nachemson A. (1976), Personal communication.

[31] Cyriax J. (1971), "Textbook of orthopaedic medicine" Vol. 2, 8th ed. (Bailliere Tindall, London.)

[32] Dalseth I. (1974), "Anatomic studies of the cranio-vertebral joints", Man. Med. 6; 130.

[33] Baddeley H. (1976), "Radiology of lumbar spinal stenosis" in: "The lumbar spine and back pain" ed. M. Jayson.

[34] Goldstein M. (Editor) (1975), "The research status of spinal manipulative therapy", US Department of Health, Education and Welfare.

[35] Wall P. D. (1977), Proceedings of FIMM Congress, Copenhagen.

[36] Mennell J. McM. (1960), "Back pain". (J. & A. Churchill Ltd., London.)

[37] Mathews J. A. (1976), "Epidurography — A technique for diagnosis and research" in: "The lumbar spine and back pain" ed. M. Jayson.

[38] Nachemson A. (1960), "Lumbar intradiscal pressure", Acta Orth. Scand. Suppl. 43.

[39] Tottle C. R. (1972), "Symposium on the painful back" Royal Coll. Phys., London.

[40] Fielding J. W. (1979), Quoting Rothman, R. at Orthopaedic and Physical Therapy Seminar, University of Cincinatti Medical Center, Sept. 1979.

[41] Kelly P., and Schneider G. (1975), "Manual correction of scoliosis", Proceedings of Australian Physiotherapy Congress.

[42] Tucker W. E. (1960), Active Alerted Posture. London. Livingstone.

[43] Hickey D. S., and Hukins D. W. L. (1980), "Relation Between the Structure of the Annulus Fibrosus and the Function and Failure of the Intervertebral Disc". Spine Vol. 5. No. 2. 106.

[44] White A. A., and Panjabi M. M. (1978), "Clinical Biomechanics of the Spine". J. B. Lippincott Co.

[45] Burkart S. (1980), Proceedings of IFOMT Congress. Christchurch, New Zealand.

[46] Markolf K. L., and Morris J. M. (1974), The structural components of the intervertebral disc. J.B. J.S. 56A. 675.

[47] Markolf K. L. (1972), Deformation of the thoraic lumbar intervertebral joint in response to external loads: a biomechanical study using autopsy material. J.B. J.S. 54A. 511.

[48] Salter R. (1979), Paper presented Canadian Royal College of Physicians and Surgeons Montreal.

DATE DUE

OCT 19 1994		
~~4/16/14~~	APR 2 9 2009	
DEC 1997		
MAY 0 7 2003		
OCT 0 6 2005		

Demco, Inc. 38-293